Myopathies

Library of Congress Cataloging in Publication Data

Bethlem, J
    Myopathies.

    Includes index.
    1.   Muscles––Diseases.   I.   Title.
RC925.B47   616.7′4   77-4770

Elsevier/North-Holland ISBN: 0–7204–0641–2
Lippincott ISBN: 0–397–58227–7

Publishers
Elsevier/North-Holland Biomedical Press
335 Jan van Galenstraat, POBox 211
Amsterdam The Netherlands

Sole distributors for the USA and Canada
J.B. Lippincott Company
E. Washington Sq.
Philadelphia, Pa. 19105, USA

Printed in The Netherlands

Myopathies

Jaap Bethlem MD
Professor of Neurology
University of Amsterdam

J.B. Lippincott Company
Philadelphia and Toronto

To Jaappieter

Contents

contents

Acknowledgements

I would like to express my gratitude to

King and Wala
friendship and inspiration

Anneke de Waal
assistance

Joan Wade
language

Frans Jennekens
discussions

Otto Treumann
book design

Prinses Beatrix Fonds
financial support

Introduction

When confronted with a patient suffering from a neuromuscular disease, most clinicians feel the necessity to know more on the subject of myology. Moreover, they often feel uncertain, because their knowledge, gathered as a student, is out-dated, and most of the modern and recent knowledge is scattered in a vast amount of literature, not easily or immediately at hand. This book is meant for all those clinicians, i.e. general physicians, neurologists, paediatricians, orthopaedists or specialists for rehabilitation, who recognize these feelings. It covers the most important primary disorders of muscle, and consequently only deals with a small part of the field of myology.

One of the major problems in connection with myology is the classification of the myopathies. This would often appear impossible, inconsequent or at least illogical. To overcome these disadvantages, it was first decided to present the myopathies in this book in alphabetical order. This utmost non-classification, however, only added to the confusion instead of reducing it. Therefore the disorders of muscle are given in accordance with a slightly modified version of the original classification prepared by the Research Group on Neuromuscular Diseases for the World Federation of Neurology. Although aware of the inevitable deficiencies in the above classification, it was considered better to use this rather than formulate a new one, and thereby introduce new names, new inconsequences and new misunderstandings.

This book was written for the clinician and therefore mainly gives clinical information based on the most relevant and recent publications. Putting forward personal ideas has been avoided, although the choice of the literature reviewed is in itself a personal contribution.

Myology is a fast-growing and fascinating specialism. It is to be hoped that by reading this book the clinician will become interested in this specialism, and finally absorbed by it, like the many research workers who — as recently as the last 15 years — have made myology what it is to-day.

Muscular dystrophies

The muscular dystrophies belong to the oldest known group of neuromuscular diseases, and even to-day the name muscular dystrophy is used
by some authors as an equivalent for myopathy. Well known neurologists
in the beginning of this century classified the muscular dystrophies according to the distribution of the muscular weakness. To-day, there is still no
better alternative for the classification of this genetically determined group
of disorders which have little, if anything, in common.
In none of these diseases is the primary biochemical lesion known. They
differ not only in clinical expression and rate of progression, but also from
the pathological and genetic points of view. Historical ties seem to be one
of the major reasons holding them together.

The following diseases are generally accepted as belonging to the muscular
dystrophies:
X-linked recessive muscular dystrophy or Duchenne disease (page 2).
X-linked recessive muscular dystrophy, benign or Becker type (page 26).
Facioscapulohumeral muscular dystrophy (page 29).
Scapulo-peroneal myopathies (page 33).
Distal myopathies (page 51).
Progressive external ophthalmoplegia (page 58).

In addition there is a variety of neuromuscular disorders in which there is
mainly weakness of the muscles of the proximal limbs and of the shoulder
and pelvic girdles. These diseases form the limb-girdle syndrome (page
42).

Duchenne muscular dystrophy is an X-linked recessive myopathy also named progressive muscular dystrophy, dystrophia musculorum progressiva, Duchenne disease or Duchenne de Boulogne disease. The latter name is mainly used in the French literature.

In rare instances girls with Turner syndrome may suffer from Duchenne muscular dystrophy [33,100]. Although there are reports of malignant autosomal recessive myopathies in girls [24,36,51] it is better to avoid the eponym Duchenne in these cases.

The first symptoms are usually detected by the parents when the boy starts to walk. There is indisposition to walk, difficulty with running, proneness to fall and clumsiness in getting up when lying on the floor. When the parents have already had a child with Duchenne disease they are often able to recognize the disease in the next child at a very early stage. On the other hand, some parents are convinced that their child manifested a normal motor development during the first two or three years of life, or even longer.

The disease is characterized by a progressive muscular weakness and wasting, starting in the extensors of the hip and knee joints and spreading to the extensors of the feet. This is followed by involvement of the muscles of the shoulder girdle, the upper arms and the flexors of the neck. Finally, most muscles become weak, including the intercostal and facial muscles. The calf muscles may remain strong for many years. When these muscles become affected there is often enlargement due to replacement of the muscle fibres by connective and fatty tissues. This pseudo-hypertrophy is not only seen in the calf muscles, but may also be present in the deltoids, infraspinati, triceps, quadriceps and gluteal muscles.

The patient has a waddling, lordotic gait, and a protruding abdomen. There is a tendency to walk on his toes and to place his feet far apart. When he is asked to stand up from the lying position, he often turns on his side and is only able to reach a standing position when he uses his hands. He usually puts his hands on his knees and then 'climbs up' his upper legs in order to stand upright (Gower's sign). Accordingly, he is not able to stand up from a chair without using his arms. When climbing stairs, he likes to crawl on his hands and feet or he peels himself up on the bannister.

The findings, present in a very early state of the disease, can be summarized as follows [89]: hip waddle on walking fast or running, hesitation for balance when ascending stairs, the need to shift the weight a little to one side in order to rise from the seated position, the impossibility to perform a standing jump, and the presence of flat feet secondary to tight heel cords. The tendon reflexes are diminished or absent, except for the ankle reflexes which can be elicited even in an advanced stage of the disease.

At the age of five or six years, the muscular growth outstrips the muscular breakdown and gives rise to an apparent stand-still or even improvement of the condition. There is, however, steady progression, and a few years later the patient is unable to walk without support and is confined to a wheel-chair. This weakness is often accelerated by the development of contractures (calves, hamstrings, hip flexors) or by bedrest, for instance, as a result of a febrile illness, injury or operation (often an orthopaedic surgical procedure).

Once the patient is confined to a wheel-chair, kyphoscoliosis and fixed flexion of the knee and elbow joints are likely to occur. Many boys become very obese due to immobility, but in the final stage of the disease extreme emaciation may be seen. Skeletal deformities and severe decalcification are the result of the muscular weakness [101] and may lead to liability of the bones to fracture.

Pulmonary problems are frequently encountered in advanced stages of the disease [13,88].

Death occurs usually between the ages of 15 and 20 and results from pneumonia or cardiac failure.

Cardiac manifestations

Cardiac involvement is extremely common and thought to be present in over 80 per cent of the patients. Electrocardiographic changes are noted during all stages of the disease, even when overt clinical evidence of heart disease is lacking [26]. The most common findings consist of tall right precordial R waves and/or deep left precordial Q waves [28,91,102]. Enlargement of the heart, congestive heart failure and various cardiac dysrhythmias, including sinus tachycardia, may occur in the advanced stages [54].

Pathology of the heart muscle may show fibrous bands, particularly present in the left ventricle and the left side of the interventricular septum [97].

Intellectual changes

Mental retardation is present in 30–50 per cent of the patients. The mean IQ ratings vary in different series, but IQs range from about 50 to 90 in most patients in whom intellectual impairment is present. Verbal and performance IQs are equally affected. The mental subnormality is present from birth and is non-progressive. It is not significantly influenced by psychological, social or educational consequences of the muscle disablement, nor is it dependent on the duration or severity of the muscular involvement. This has been confirmed in studies of children with severe locomotor disability due to spinal muscular atrophy and with similar social backgrounds. These children showed a normal mental development.

In families containing two or more patients, the affected members often have a similar IQ, suggesting that mental retardation may be genetically determined [16,53].

Electroencephalographic abnormalities are frequently present but are unrelated to the mental development or to the severity of the disease.

The weight of the brain is within the normal range, while no histological abnormalities related to the presence of mental retardation are present [25].

Electromyography

The electromyogram shows reduction in mean duration of small amplitude motor unit potentials and increase in polyphasic forms. A full interference pattern is found during only slight or moderate contraction. These brief, small, abundant motor unit action potentials (BSAP pattern) cannot be accepted as diagnostic proof of Duchenne disease or any other myopathy [31].

Laboratory findings

There is almost no neuromuscular disease in which such extremely high serum creatine phosphokinase (CPK) activities may be present. Therefore, this laboratory finding is very important and a sensitive index for the diagnosis of Duchenne muscular dystrophy.

CPK activity is already raised directly after birth and may increase after that, even when the patient is still in a preclinical stage of disease. There is a tendency to a steady decrease of the serum CPK activity as the duration of the disease increases [40,96]. It has been shown that the MB isoenzyme of CPK was markedly elevated in the serum early in the course of the disease and that the probable source is skeletal, not cardiac muscle [90].

The testing of the activity of serum pyruvate kinase (PK) also revealed a very high sensitivity [2]. The activities of other serum enzymes, i.e. aldolase, lactate dehydrogenase, glutamic oxalacetic transaminase (GOT) and glutamic pyruvic transaminase (GPT), may also be increased, but these findings are less consistent, and their testing consequently of less diagnostic value than that of CPK and PK activities.

A marked creatinuria is often present in Duchenne disease, but this is a non-specific finding seen in many unrelated neuromuscular disorders.

In the muscle tissue, a significant and selective, moderate decrease of glyoxalase I activity was found [48]. A large number of other biochemical abnormalities have been reported, but the exact mechanism or the significance of these findings is at present difficult to evaluate.

Muscle pathology

Muscle biopsies show a marked variation in muscle fibre diameter, necrotic fibres, phagocytosis, and regenerating basophilic fibres with vesicular nuclei and prominent nucleoli. These structural changes are often seen in small foci.

Another constant finding are swollen, rounded fibres, scattered throughout the tissue. They contain homogenic eosinophilic material (hyaline fibres) and stain darker than the other fibres with most staining techniques. Many authors consider these dark fibres as artifacts; nevertheless, they agree that their incidence is very consistent in Duchenne muscular dystrophy. Although it is not always possible to recognize all muscle fibre types, there does not appear to be any selective fibre type involvement. However, comparison of the published data of the literature is difficult because different systems of muscle fibre typing are used. As a rule the myofibrillar ATPase reaction at pH 9.4 is the best technique to differentiate fibre types. When other staining methods were used, such as NADH, SDH and phosphorylase stains, more information could be obtained and a marked increase of intermediate staining fibres was observed [8].

An increase in the number of internal nuclei may be found, but it is never a prominent feature. A considerable increase in nuclear size has been observed, although the significance of this finding is not clear [98].

Exhaustive investigations of the muscle spindle showed various degenerative changes and atrophy of the intrafusal muscle fibres without evidence of regeneration. There was a trend for spindles, in severely affected muscles, to contain fewer intrafusal muscle fibres than spindles in normal or moderately affected muscles. Replacement of the spindle and its capsule by a fibrous scar was seen in advanced stages [92].

A marked proliferation of endomysial and perimysial connective tissue and, in later stages, an increase of fatty tissue, is seen in all cases, while cellular infiltrates are often present.

Ultrastructural changes are completely non-specific; a marked increase of satellite cells is a consistent finding [99].

Pathogenesis
There are at present three main hypotheses concerning the pathogenesis of Duchenne disease, i.e. the vascular, the neurogenic and the myogenic hypothesis.

The vascular hypothesis. For many years Démos and his co-workers have postulated that Duchenne disease was basically a disorder of the muscle microcirculation [20–23]. Arguments in favour of this theory were the following findings in the patients: early appearance of vasomotor disorders of the extremities, early development (in some cases preclinical) of abnormalities in the arm-to-arm circulation time, low muscle blood flow at high work loads and low oxygen consumption, the decrease of blood platelet diphenoloxidases (enzymes which may play part in the inactivation of catacholamines) and finally the beneficial effect of vasodilator treatment. Moreover, in the female carriers they found an abnormally high frequency of Raynaud syndrome (59 per cent), and a decrease in the peripheral circulation time (50 per cent).

On histopathological grounds, i.e. the presence of foci consisting of grouped muscle fibres undergoing necrosis or regeneration, W.K. Engel and his co-workers suggested that an ischaemic mechanism played a role in the pathogenesis of the muscular changes [32]. Similar focal histopathological abnormalities could be produced in rabbits by microarterial embolization [39], and in rats by the combination of aortic ligation and 5-hydroxytryptamine (serotonin) injections [60] or by the combination of injections of serotonin and imipramine, a pharmacological agent blocking uptake of biogenic amines into platelets [73].

A significant defect in the initial uptake of serotonin by platelets was found, raising the possibility of a defect in the metabolism of biogenic amines [70]. Urinary excretion of catacholamines and indoleamines was normal, suggesting that the muscle lesions did not result from a simple excess of circulating biogenic amines [61].

Other investigators found no sufficient evidence of a structural or functional defect in the microcirculation to support the vascular hypothesis: Xenon clearance studies revealed no abnormalities in muscle blood flow [12,74]. Light and electron microscopic studies showed no abnormalities of the arterioles, capillaries or venules [52]. No relevant changes of the small arterial vessels and capillaries were seen by light microscopy, although thin basement membranes of the capillaries were observed at the ultrastructural level [71]. The mean muscle fibre area served per capillary was essentially normal [46]. Although the mean capillary size was found to be significantly increased and two-thirds of the capillaries had replicated basal lamina, these abnormalities were not considered as adequate morphological evidence in favour of the vascular hypothesis.

Statistical analysis of the groups of fibres undergoing active necrosis and phagocytosis showed a slightly greater number of groups of four or more of such fibres than might otherwise be expected by chance. Moreover, 70 per cent of the necrotic fibres occurred in isolation [12]. Experimentally induced ischaemic lesions in rat muscles also showed significant dissimilarity with the lesions in Duchenne disease [49].

The neurogenic hypothesis. In 1971 McComas and his co-workers developed a new electromyographic technique involving incrementing nerve–muscle stimulation. They found a marked reduction in the number of functioning motor units in the extensor digitorum brevis muscle of Duchenne patients [57]. This was attributed to 'sick' motor neurones that had difficulty in maintaining satisfactory synaptic connections with muscle fibres [56].

Other electrophysiological studies have failed to confirm these observations [7,72].

The total number of limb motor neurons in the anterior horns of the lumbosacral spinal cord in Duchenne disease was found to be normal [97]. The terminal innervation ratio (i.e. the number of muscle fibres innervated by a given number of terminal motor arborizations) was also normal [14,15].

Electron microscopy of the motor end-plates showed a focal atrophy of the post-synaptic folds [47] and separation of the end-plate terminals from the sole plate [38]. The mean nerve terminal area, the mitochondrial area per nerve terminal, the synaptic vesicle count per unit nerve terminal area and the synaptic vesicle diameter were normal [47]. No degenerating nerve terminals or intramuscular nerves were observed. Therefore, no morphological evidence for the neurogenic hypothesis could be established. Finally, it has been shown that this hypothesis is not compatible with the decline with age of serum CPK activity in carriers [96].

There is also a 'neurovascular' hypothesis suggesting that abnormal function of sympathetic vasomotor neurons leads to functional ischaemia in active muscles [3].

The myogenic hypothesis. Many studies have been carried out in search of a basic abnormality in the muscle cell itself. Mainly quantitative alterations of myofibrillary proteins, such as actin, myosin, tropomyosin and troponin, were found and these are probably secondary to the disease [34,85]. An increase in protein synthesis by muscle polyribosomes was present in Duchenne disease and in the carriers of the defective gene [43,44].

Recent investigations suggest that in Duchenne disease there is an abnormal permeability of muscle cell membrane. This membrane abnormality was already assumed by the finding of increased activities of sarcoplasmic enzymes in the serum, although none of these proved to be specific.

Some biochemical abnormalities of the sarcotubular membranes were consistently found by many others, such as a low initial and total calcium uptake [79,86,87,93]. The phospholipid and cholesterol contents of the sarcoplasmic reticulum were normal, but the proportions of individual phospholipids were altered, with a marked decrease of phosphatidylcholine. However, it has been suggested that contamination of the membrane fraction by microsomes from fat and connective tissues could account for the abnormal lipid composition and for the deficient calcium binding.

In non-necrotic muscle fibres, one or more wedge-shaped lesions ('delta lesions'), with the base resting on the fibre surface, were seen [65]. The inner plasma membrane overlying this lesion was either absent or disrupted, but the outer basal lamina was always preserved. Exposure of biopsy specimens to peroxidase-containing extracellular fluid showed focal penetration of peroxidase in areas, closely corresponding in size, shape and frequency to those of the delta lesions. These findings were considered as an early and possible basic abnormality in the plasma membrane of the muscle fibres in Duchenne disease, but other authorities think of them as artifacts.

A more generalized membrane defect in Duchenne disease is suggested by several abnormalities of the erythrocyte membranes. There is a significant increase in the rate of phosphorylation of the erythrocyte spectrin peak II [80]. Abnormal lipid composition and abnormal enzymatic activities have been found [4,59,81], as well as reduced deformability [77]. In both patients and carriers morphological changes of the red blood cells were seen with the scanning electron microscope [63].

Carrier detection

Because no effective treatment is known for Duchenne muscular dystrophy, genetic counselling is very important in this X-linked recessive disease.

When a woman, who is a known carrier for the gene for Duchenne disease, is pregnant, there are four possibilities: she will have either a girl who is normal, a girl who is a carrier, a boy who is normal or a boy suffering from Duchenne disease. To rule out the possibility of her giving birth to a boy, antenatal sex determination by amniocentesis can be carried out, with selective abortion of male foetuses. One of the disadvantages of this procedure is that the incidence of carriers will be expected to increase linearly with each generation, since sons will be replaced by daughters, half of whom will be carriers [29]. Moreover, the new-born girl, who is a carrier, will be confronted later in her life with exactly the same problem as her mother.

At present, one of the main problems is the impossibility of recognizing all carriers because there is no method available that can detect one hundred per cent of the cases.

Duchenne carriers are classified as follows:

Definite carrier: the mother of an affected son with either an affected brother, maternal uncle, sister's son, one or more affected grandsons or other male relative in the female line of inheritance;

Probable carrier: the mother of two or more affected sons, but no other known affected relatives;

Possible carrier: the mother with only one affected son and no other affected male relatives; or a female without an affected son, but with a male relative with the disease, such as a brother, the son of a sister, maternal uncle or maternal cousin.

Daughters of a definite or probable carrier and a female related to a definite carrier, have a known statistical risk of being a carrier.

Female relatives, other than daughters, of a probable carrier, and the mother, sister or other female relative of an isolated case, have an unknown statistical risk of being a carrier [95].
The following methods are at present available for carrier detection:

1. Physical examination. The presence of clinical symptoms and manifestations of muscular weakness in a small proportion (approximately 5 per cent) of heterozygotes has been attributed to inactivation mainly of the X-chromosome bearing the normal gene in early embryonic development (Lyon hypothesis [55]). However, random X-inactivation is not sufficient to explain the large proportion of manifesting carriers within one and the same family. Additional, possibly genetic, regulatory mechanisms are therefore likely to exist [67].

Many manifesting carriers present with a slowly progressive myopathy that predominantly affects the muscles of the lower limbs and the pelvic girdle.

Some carriers may show pseudo-hypertrophic calf muscles, but no progression is noticed in these women. It has been postulated that careful and detailed manual muscle testing can reveal weakness in several proximal muscles [82]; this was found in 19 of 21 mothers of patients. Most of these women had no symptomatic complaints and apparently the detectable weakness had made no appreciable difference in their daily activities.

2. Determination of serum creatine phosphokinase (CPK) activity. With this method about 60–80 per cent of the definite and probable carriers can be detected [42,58,68,83]. Consequently, a normal serum CPK activity does not rule out the possibility of the tested woman being a carrier. There seems to be no value in determining the CPK level following exercise, but it is recommended that at least three or four separate estimations of the activity of this enzyme in the serum should be performed [78].

The level of the serum CPK activity in known carriers tends to decline with age [69]. Therefore, very young sisters of affected boys should be tested and one should not wait until they have grown up. Also, there is a decline during early pregnancy. This is also found in normal pregnant women, and thus the CPK levels of a potential carrier should be compared with values obtained in pregnant women at a comparable period of gestation [50]. Probability calculations, based upon the exact levels of serum CPK activity, even when within normal range, may also be helpful in genetic counselling [30]. So far, the level of the serum CPK activity seems to be one of the most reliable indexes of the carrier state [37], while the estimation has the advantage of being a routine procedure that can be carried out in every laboratory.

3. Determination of serum pyruvate kinase (PK) activity. It is probable that the elevation of the activity of serum PK in carriers is more sensitive than that of serum CPK [2].

4. Determination of serum haemopexin. By immunoelectrophoretic investigations of blood serum proteins in carriers, Askanas [5,6] found an additional line in the fraction of β_1 globulins corresponding to haemopexin. The level of haemopexin concentration in the serum was found to be significantly higher in definite, probable and possible carriers with a raised serum CPK activity [17]. In 33 per cent of the possible carriers with a normal CPK activity, there was also an abnormal haemopexin level. The concomitant use of this method and the determination of the serum CPK activity, raised the percentage of detection of definite and probable carriers to 87 per cent [18].

5. Determination of serum LDH isoenzymes. An increase of LDH 1 and 2 isoenzymes, with concomitant decrease of LDH 3–5, was thought to be diagnostic for carriers [41]. On the other hand, the total serum LDH activity was consistently found to be normal in all carriers.

6. Erythrocyte peak II phosphorylation. A significant increase of the mean value of the endogenous phosphorylation of one of the major protein peaks of the erythrocyte membrane was found in mothers of patients [82]. However, individual carriers cannot be evaluated solely by this method, since the values for individual carriers extensively overlap the normal range.

7. Scanning electron microscopy of erythrocytes. Unmanipulated erythrocytes show a large increased percentage of cup-shaped red blood cells (stomatocytes) when examined by scanning electron microscopy. So far, this was found in all the examined definite, probable and possible carriers, without false-negative results. However, false-positive results occurred in about 5 per cent of controls, so that this method alone cannot be used for the detection of carriers [63].

8. Elastimetry of erythrocytes. Based on the observations of abnormalities in surface contour as seen by scanning electron microscopy, the membrane elasticity of the red blood cells was tested using cell elastimetry [62]. Using a method in which negative pressure aspiration of the erythrocytes was measured, a significant reduction in deformability of the erythrocyte membrane was found in known carriers [77].

9. Direct macrophage inhibition test. Cellular hypersensitivity to muscle tissue, examined with a direct macrophage inhibition test [94], was found to be present in the lymphocytes of some carriers [64].

10. Determination of total body potassium. Slight but significant reduction in body potassium concentration and a reduced biological half-life of rubidium chloride Rb 86, was reported in some carriers [9,10]. However, other authors considered these findings to have no great value in carrier detection [11].

11. Muscle pathology. In a proportion of carriers light and electron microscopy of a muscle biopsy may show abnormalities [1,45,75,84]. These include focal necrosis and phagocytosis, large 'dark' fibres, basophilic fibres with vesicular nuclei and prominent nucleoli, and an increase in the number of fibres with internal nuclei. Central nuclear counts in biopsy specimens of the rectus abdominis muscles and the application of Bayes' theorem, seemed to be a useful means of discriminating between carriers and non-carriers [19].

Ultrastructural alterations include focal myofilamentous loss, streaming of the Z discs, subsarcolemmal collections of mitochondria, and dilatation of the elements of the sarcoplasmic reticulum.

12. Muscle protein synthesis. High amino acid incorporation of polyribosomes was found in 42 of 63 definite, probable and possible carriers [44]. The increase in protein synthesis in 25 of these carriers also involved high collagen formation. This was especially seen in carriers under 34 years of age. Concomitant use of muscle ribosomal protein synthesis with determination of the activity of serum CPK, can raise the identification of carriers to more than 90 per cent.

13. Muscle LDH isoenzymes. An abnormal lactate dehydrogenase isoenzyme pattern in the muscle tissue, i.e. a decrease in the slow migrating LDH 5 fraction, has been found in some carriers [41,76].

14. Muscle troponin activity. Troponin activity of natural actomyosin isolated from muscle tissue, showed greatly decreased values in Duchenne disease and also a slightly decreased value in one of two carriers [34].

15. Electromyography. Quantitative electromyography with measurement of the age-corrected mean action potential duration, the number of phases per potential or the proportion of polyphasic potentials, may be an useful method for identifying carriers [35]. Automatic methods of quantitating EMG changes, based on the ratio of action potentials duration to the number of phases per potential, also showed a significant rise of this ratio in some of the carriers [66]. The detection percentage can be improved when combined with determination of serum CPK activity.

16. Electrocardiography. On inspection most carriers show no changes in their electrocardiogram. However, careful measurement of the R and S wave in V_1, showed that the algebraic sum of these waves was significantly greater in carriers than in normal women [27].

References 1 Afifi,A.K.,Bergman,R.A.,Zellweger,H.
A possible role for electron microscopy in detection of carriers of Duchenne type muscular dystrophy.
J.Neurol.Neurosurg.Psychiat.1973,36: 643–650

2 Alberts,M.C.,Samaha,F.J.
Serum pyruvate kinase in muscle disease and carrier states.
Neurology(Minneap.)1974,24:462–464

3 Appenzeller,O.
Pathogenesis of muscular dystrophies. Sympathetic neurovascular components.
Arch.Neurol.(Chic.)1975,32:2–4

4 Araki,S.,Mawatari,S.
Ouabain and erythrocyte-ghost adenosine triphosphatase. Effects in human muscular dystrophies.
Arch.Neurol.(Chic.)1971,24:187–190

5 Askanas,W.
Identification of the agent responsible for the abnormal immunoelectrophoretic pattern of serum in Duchenne's progressive muscular dystrophy.
Life Sci.1966,5:1767–1773

6 Askanas,W.
Immunoelectrophoretic investigations of blood serum proteins in muscular diseases.
J.Neurol.Neurosurg.Psychiat.1967,30:43–46

7 Ballantyne,J.P.,Hansen,S.
Myopathies: the neurogenic hypothesis.
Lancet 1974,I:1060–1061

8 Baloh,R.,Cancilla,P.A.
An appraisal of histochemical fiber types in Duchenne muscular dystrophy.
Neurology(Minneap.)1972,22:1243–1252

9 Blahd,W.H.,Cassen,B.,Lederer,M.

Decreased body potassium in nondystrophic relatives of
patients with muscular dystrophy.
New Engl.J.Med.1964,270:197–198

10   Blahd,W.H.,Lederer,M.,Cassen,B.
The significance of decreased body potassium concentrations
in patients with muscular dystrophy and nondystrophic
relatives.
New Engl.J.Med.1967,276:1349–1352

11   Bradley,W.G.,Gardner-Medwin,D.,Haggith,J.,Walton,J.N.,
Hesp,R.
Duchenne muscular dystrophy. Use of rubidium chloride
Rb 86 in the detection of carriers of the gene.
Arch.Neurol.(Chic.)1971,25:193–197

12   Bradley,W.G.,O'Brien,M.D.,Walder,D.N.,Murchison,D.,
Johnson,M.,Newell,D.J.
Failure to confirm a vascular cause of muscular dystrophy.
Arch.Neurol.(Chic.)1975,32:466–473

13   Burke,S.S.,Grove,N.M.,Houser,C.R.,Johnson,D.M.
Respiratory aspects of pseudohypertrophic muscular
dystrophy.
Amer.J.Dis.Child.1971,121:230–236

14   Coërs,C.,Telerman-Toppet,N.,Gérard,J.-M.
Terminal innervation ratio in neuromuscular disease.
I. Methods and controls.
Arch.Neurol.(Chic.)1973,29:210–214.

15   Coërs,C.,Telerman-Toppet,N.,Gérard,J.-M.
Terminal innervation ratio in neuromuscular disease.
II. Disorders of lower motor neuron, peripheral nerve, and
muscle.
Arch.Neurol.(Chic.)1973,29:215–222

16   Cohen,H.J.,Molnar,G.E.,Taft,L.T.
The genetic relationship of progressive muscular dystrophy
(Duchenne type) and mental retardation.
Develop.Med.Child Neurol.1968,10:754–765

17   Danieli,G.A.,Angelini,C.
Duchenne carrier detection.
Lancet 1976,II:90

18   Danieli,G.A.,Angelini,C.
Duchenne carrier detection.

Lancet 1976,II:415–416

19   DeChairBaker,W.,Morgan,G.,Stark,A.
     Central nuclear counting in detection of carriers of Duchenne
     type muscular dystrophy.
     In:Clinical Studies in Myology.Proceedings of the 2nd
     International Congress on Muscle Diseases,Perth,
     22–26 November 1971.Part 2.B.A.Kakulus(ed.).
     Amsterdam,Excerpta Medica,1973,pp.648–652.(Int.Congr.
     Ser.295).

20   Démos,J.
     Mesure des temps de circulation chez 79 myopathes. Etude
     statistique des résultats. Rôle du degré de l'atteinte
     musculaire clinique, du mode évolutif de la maladie,
     du sexe du malade, des saisons.
     Rev.franç.Etud.clin.biol.1961,6:876–887

21   Démos,J.
     Early diagnosis and treatment of rapidly developing Duchenne
     de Boulogne type myopathy (type DDB I).
     Amer.J.phys.Med.1971,50:271–284

22   Démos,J.
     Platelet diphenoloxidases in progressive muscular dystrophy
     (P.M.D.).
     Clin.Genet.1973,4:79–90

23   Démos,J.,Place,T.,Chereau,H.
     Myopathy – a disorder of the microcirculation?
     In:Muscle Diseases,J.N.Walton,N.Canal and G.Scarlato
     (eds.).Amsterdam,Excerpta Medica,1970,pp.408–411
     (Int.Congr.Ser.199)

24   Dubowitz,V.
     Progressive muscular dystrophy of the Duchenne type in
     females and its mode of inheritance.
     Brain 1960,83:432–439

25   Dubowitz,V.,Crome,L.
     The central nervous system in Duchenne muscular dystrophy.
     Brain 1969,92:805–808

26   Durnin,R.E.,Ziska,J.H.,Zellweger,H.
     Observations on the electrocardiogram in Duchenne's
     progressive muscular dystrophy.
     Helv.paediat.Acta 1971,26:331–339

27 Emery,A.E.H.
Abnormalities of the electrocardiogram in female carriers of
Duchenne muscular dystrophy.
Brit.med.J.1969,2:418–420

28 Emery,A.E.H.
Abnormalities of the electrocardiogram in hereditary
myopathies.
J.med.Genet.1972,9:8–12

29 Emery,A.E.H.
The aetiology of polymyositis. Discussion.
In:Clinical Studies in Myology.Proceedings of the
2nd International Congress on Muscle Diseases,Perth,
22–26 November 1971.Part 2 by B.A.Kakulas(ed.).
Amsterdam,Excerpta Medica,1973,pp.36–38.
(Int.Congr.Ser.295)

30 Emery,A.E.H.,Morton,R.
Genetic counselling in lethal x-linked disorders.
Acta genet.(Basel)1968,18:534–542

31 Engel,W.K.
Brief, small, abundant motor-unit action potentials. A further
critique of electromyographic interpretation.
Neurology(Minneap.)1975,25:173–176

32 Engel,W.K.
The vascular hypothesis.
In:Recent Advances in Myology.Proceedings of the
3rd International Congress on Muscle Diseases,
Newcastle upon Tyne,15–21September,1974.
W.G.Bradley,D.Gardner-Medwin,J.N.Walton(eds.).
Amsterdam,Excerpta Medica,1975,pp.166–177.
(Int.Congr.Ser.360)

33 Ferrier,P.,Bamatter,F.,Klein,D.
Muscular dystrophy (Duchenne) in a girl with Turner's
syndrome.
J.med.Genet.1965,2:38–46

34 Furukawa,T.,Peter,J.B.
Muscular dystrophy and other myopathies. Troponin
activity of natural actomyosin from skeletal muscle.
Arch.Neurol.(Chic.)1972,26:385–390

35 Gardner-Medwin,D.

Studies of the carrier in the Duchenne type of muscular
dystrophy. 2. Quantitative electromyography as a method
of carrier detection.
J.Neurol.Neurosurg.Psychiat.1968,31:124–134

36 Gardner-Medwin,D.
Muscular dystrophy in young girls.
Brit.med.J.1970,4:51–52

37 Gardner-Medwin,D.,Pennington,R.J.,Walton,J.N.
The detection of carriers of X-linked muscular dystrophy genes.
A review of some methods studied in Newcastle upon Tyne.
J.neurol.Sci.1971,13:459–474

38 Harriman,D.G.F.
A comparison of the fine structure of motor end-plates
in Duchenne dystrophy and in human neurogenic diseases.
J.neurol.Sci.1976,28:233–247

39 Hathaway,P.W.,Engel,W.K.,Zellweger,H.
Experimental myopathy after microarterial embolization.
Comparison with childhood x-linked pseudohypertrophic
muscular dystrophy.
Arch.Neurol.(Chic.)1970,22:365–378

40 Heyck, H., Laudahn,G.
Fermentchemische Serumbefunde bei Myopathien.
In:Myopathien.Genetik,Biochemie,Pathologie,Klinik und
Therapie unter besonderer Berücksichtigung des Kindesalters.
R.Beckmann(ed.).Stuttgart,Thieme,1965,pp.176–187

41 Hooshmand,H.,Dove,J.,Suter,C.
The use of serum lactate dehydrogenase isoenzymes in
the diagnosis of muscle diseases.
Neurology(Minneap.)1969,19:26–31

42 Hughes,R.C.,Park,D.C.,Parsons,M.E.,O'Brien,M.D.
Serum creatine kinase studies in the detection of carriers
of Duchenne dystrophy.
J.Neurol.Neurosurg.Psychiat.1971,34:527–530

43 Ionasescu,V.,Zellweger,H.,Conway,T.W.
Ribosomal protein synthesis in Duchenne muscular dystrophy.
Arch.Biochem.Biophys.1971,144:51–58

44 Ionasescu,V.,Zellweger,H.,Shirk,P.,Conway,T.W.
Identification of carriers of Duchenne muscular dystrophy
by muscle protein synthesis.

Neurology(Minneap.)1973,23:497–502

45 Ionescu,V.,Radu,H.,Nicolescu,P.
Identification of Duchenne muscular dystrophy carriers:
electron microscopical investigation of skeletal muscle.
Arch.Path.1975,99:436–441

46 Jerusalem,F.,Engel,A.G.,Gomez,M.R.
Duchenne dystrophy. I. Morphometric study of the muscle
microvasculature.
Brain 1974,97:115–122

47 Jerusalem,F.,Engel,A.G.,Gomez,M.R.
Duchenne dystrophy. II. Morphometric study of motor
end-plate fine structure.
Brain 1974,97:123–130

48 Kar,N.C.,Pearson,C.M.
Glyoxalase enzyme system in human muscular dystrophy.
Clin.chim.Acta 1975,65:153–155

49 Karpati,G.,Carpenter,S.,Melmed,C.,Eisen,A.A.
Experimental ischemic myopathy.
J.neurol.Sci.1974,23:129–161

50 King,B.,Spikesman,A.,Emery,A.E.H.
The effect of pregnancy on serum levels of creatine kinase.
Clin.chim.Acta 1972,35:267–269

51 Kloepfer,H.W.,Talley,C.
Autosomal recessive inheritance of Duchenne type muscular
dystrophy.
Ann.hum.Genet.1958,22:138–143

52 Koehler,J.P.
Blood vessel structure in Duchenne muscular dystrophy.
Neurology(Minneap.)1974,24:354.

53 Kozicka,A.,Prot,J.,Wasilewski,R.
Mental retardation in patients with Duchenne progressive
muscular dystrophy.
J.neurol.Sci.1971,14:209–213

54 Leth,A.,Wulff,K.
Myocardiopathy in Duchenne progressive muscular dystrophy.
Acta paediat.scand.1976,65:28–32

55 Lyon,M.F.
Sex chromatin and gene action in the mammalian
X-chromosome.

Amer.J.hum.Genet.1962,14:135–148

56 McComas,A.J.,Sica,R.E.P.,Campbell,M.J.
'Sick' motoneurones. A unifying concept of muscle disease.
Lancet 1971,I:321–325

57 McComas,A.J.,Sica,R.E.P.,Currie,S.
An electrophysiological study of Duchenne dystrophy.
J.Neurol.Neurosurg.Psychiat.1971,34:461–468

58 McCormick,D.,Allen,I.V.
Serum creatine phosphokinase in the detection of carriers of
Duchenne's muscular dystrophy in Northern Ireland.
Ulster med.J.1976,45:79–83.

59 Nawatari,S.,Schonberg,M.,Olarte,M.
Biochemical abnormalities of erythrocyte membranes in
Duchenne dystrophy. Adenosine triphosphatase and adenyl
cyclase.
Arch.Neurol.(Chic.)1976,33:489–493

60 Mendell,J.R.,Engel,W.K.,Derrer,E.C.
Duchenne muscular dystrophy: functional ischemia
reproduces its characteristic lesions.
Science 1971,172:1143–1145

61 Mendell,J.R.,Murphy,D.L.,Engel,W.K.,Chase,T.N.,
Gordon,E.
Catecholamines and indoleamines in patients with
Duchenne muscular dystrophy.
Arch.Neurol.(Chic.)1972,27:518–520

62 Miller,M.E.
Pathology of chemotaxis and random mobility.
Seminars in Hematology,1975,12:59–82

63 Miller,S.E.,Roses,A.D.,Appel,S.H.
Scanning electron microscopy studies in muscular dystrophy.
Arch.Neurol.(Chic.)1976,33:172–174

64 Minderhoud,J.M.,Teelken,A.W.,Leenstra-Borsje,H.,
Oosten,J.K.
Cellular hypersensitivity to myelin and muscle tissue in man
examined with a direct macrophage migration inhibition test.
II. Muscle diseases.
Clin.Neurol.Neurosurg.1974,77:234–240

65 Mokri,B.,Engel,A.G.
Duchenne dystrophy: electron microscopic findings pointing

to a basic or early abnormality in the plasma membrane of the muscle fiber.
Neurology(Minneap.)1975,25:1111–1120

66   Moosa,A.,Brown,B.H.,Dubowitz,V.
Quantitative electromyography: carrier detection in Duchenne type muscular dystrophy using a new automatic technique.
J.Neurol.Neurosurg.Psychiat.1972,35:841–844

67   Moser,H.,Emery,A.E.H.
The manifesting carrier in Duchenne muscular dystrophy.
Clin.Genet.1974,5:271–284

68   Moser,H.,Mumenthaler,M.,Wiesmann,U.
Biochemical,histological and clinical findings in female carriers of progressive muscular dystrophy of the Duchenne type.
Schweiz.med.Wschr.1971,101:537–542

69   Munsat,T.L.,Baloh,R.,Pearson,C.M.,FowlerJr.W.
Serum enzyme alterations in neuromuscular disorders.
J.Amer.med.Ass.1973,226:1536–1543

70   Murphy,D.L.,Mendell,J.R.,Engel,W.K.
Serotonin and platelet function in Duchenne muscular dystrophy.
Arch.Neurol.(Chic.)1973,28:239–242

71   Musch,B.C.,Papapetropoulos,T.A.,McQueen,D.A., Hudgson,P.,Weightman,D.
A comparison of the structure of small blood vessels in normal, denervated and dystrophic human muscle.
J.neurol.Sci.1975,26:221–234

72   Panayiotopoulos,C.P.,Scarpalezos,S.,Papapetropoulos,T.
Electrophysiological estimation of motor units in Duchenne muscular dystrophy.
J.neurol.Sci.1974,23:89–98

73   Parker,J.M.,Mendell,J.R.
Proximal myopathy induced by 5-HT-imipramine simulates Duchenne dystrophy.
Nature(Lond.)1974,247:103–104

74   Paulson,O.B.,Engel,A.G.,Gomez,M.R.
Muscle blood flow in Duchenne type muscular dystrophy, limb-girdle dystrophy, polymyositis, and in normal controls.
J.Neurol.Neurosurg.Phychiat.1974,37:685–690

75   Pearce,G.W.,Pearce,J.M.S.,Walton,J.N.
The Duchenne type muscular dystrophy: histopathological
studies of the carrier state.
Brain 1966,89:109–120

76   Pearson,C.M.,Kar,N.C.
Isoenzymes: general considerations and alterations in human
and animal myopathies.
Ann.N.Y.Acad.Sci.1966,138:293–303

77   Percy,A.K.,Miller,M.E.
Reduced deformability of erythrocyte membranes from
patients with Duchenne muscular dystrophy.
Nature(Lond.)1975,258:147–148

78   Perry,T.B.,Fraser,F.C.
Variability of serum creatine phosphokinase activity in
normal women and carriers of the gene for Duchenne
muscular dystrophy.
Neurology(Minneap.)1973,23:1316–1323

79   Peter,J.B.,Worsfold,M.
Muscular dystrophy and other myopathies: sarcotubular
vesicles in early disease.
Biochem.Med.1969,2:364–371

80   Roses,A.D.,Appel,S.H.
Erythrocyte spectrin peak II phosphorylation in Duchenne
muscular dystrophy.
J.neurol.Sci.1976,29:185–193

81   Roses,A.D.,Herbstreith,M.H.,Appel,S.H.
Membrane protein kinase alteration in Duchenne muscular
dystrophy.
Nature(Lond.)1975,254:350–351

82   Roses,A.D.,Roses,M.J.,Miller,S.E.,HullJr,K.L.,Appel,S.H.
Carrier detection in Duchenne muscular dystrophy.
New Engl.J.Med.1976,294:193–198

83   Rotthauwe,H.W.,Kowalewski,S.
Identification of the carrier state in the severe recessive
X-linked muscular dystrophy (Duchenne type). I. Assay of
activated serum creatine kinase activity in serum.
Z.Kinderheilk.1973,115:333–342

84   Roy,S.,Dubowitz,V.
Carrier detection in Duchenne muscular dystrophy.

A comparative study of electron microscopy, light microscopy and serum enzymes.
J.Neurol.Sci.1970,11:65–79

85 Samaha,F.J.
Actomyosin alterations in Duchenne muscular dystrophy.
Arch.Neurol.(Chic.)1973,28:405–407

86 Samaha,F.J.,Congedo,C.Z.
Abnormalities in Duchenne dystrophic sarcoplasmic reticulum proteins.
Arch.Neurol.(Chic.)1975,32:355

87 Samaha,F.J.,Gergely,J.
Biochemical abnormalities of the sarcoplasmic reticulum in muscular dystrophy.
New Engl.J.Med.1969,280:184–188

88 Siegel,I.M.
Pulmonary problems in Duchenne muscular dystrophy.
Diagnosis, prophylaxis, and treatment.
Phys.Ther.1975,55:160–162

89 Siegel,I.M.
Very early diagnosis of Duchenne muscular dystrophy.
Lancet 1976,II:90–91

90 Silverman,L.M.,Mendell,J.R.,Sahenk,Z.,Fontana,M.B.
Significance of creatine phosphokinase isoenzymes in Duchenne dystrophy.
Neurology (Minneap.)1976,26:561–564

91 Slucka,C.
The electrocardiogram in Duchenne progressive muscular dystrophy
Circulation 1968,38:933–940

92 Swash,M.,Fox,K.P.
The pathology of the muscle spindle in Duchenne muscular dystrophy.
J.neurol.Sci.1976,29:17–32

93 Takagi,A.,Schotland,D.L.,Rowland,L.P.
Sarcoplasmic reticulum in Duchenne muscular dystrophy.
Arch.Neurol.(Chic)1973,28:380–384

94 Teelken,A.W.,Minderhoud,J.M.
A direct macrophage migration inhibition test applied in man.
Clin.exp.Immunol.1976,24:26–32

95   Thompson,M.W.,Murphy,E.G.,McAlpine,P.J.
An assessment of the creatine kinase test in the detection
of carriers of Duchenne muscular dystrophy.
J.Pediat.1967,71 : 82–93

96   Thomson,W.H.S.,Sweetin,J.C.,Elton,R.A.
The neurogenic and myogenic hypotheses in human
(Duchenne) muscular dystrophy.
Nature(Lond.)1974,249:151–152

97   Tomlinson,B.E.,Walton,J.N.,Irving,D.
Spinal cord limb motor neurons in muscular dystrophy.
J.neurol.Sci.1974,22 : 305–327

98   Vassilopoulos,D.,Lumb,E.M.,Emery,A.E.H.
Muscle nuclear size in neuromuscular disease.
J.Neurol.Neurosurg.Psychiat.1976,39:159–162

99   Wakayama,Y.
Electron microscopic study on the satellite cell in the
muscle of Duchenne muscular dystrophy.
J.Neuropath.exp.Neurol.1976,35:532–540

100 Walton,J.N.
The inheritance of muscular dystrophy.
Acta genet.(Basel)1957,7:318

101 Walton,J.N.,Warrick,C.K.
Osseous changes in myopathy.
Brit.J.Radiol.1954,27 : 1–15

102 Zellweger,H.,Durnin,R.,Simpson,J.
The diagnostic significance of serum enzymes and
electrocardiogram in various muscular dystrophies.
Acta neurol.scand.1972,48:87–101

One of the first descriptions of an X-linked and relatively benign type of muscular dystrophy was given in 1937 by Kostakow and Derix [6], but the recognition of this disease as an entity that had to be separated from the more severe Duchenne disease was made by Becker [1,2].

The onset of the disease is between 5–20 years of age. The initial weakness is present in the muscles of the pelvic girdle and upper legs. In this stage, pseudo-hypertrophy of the calf muscles may often be seen.

After 5–10 years, manifestations of weakness of the muscles of the shoulder girdle and upper arms occur. There is gradual progression of the weakness and wasting, including the distal muscles of the extremities. In some families, equinovarus contractures and flexion contractures of the elbows may develop in a relatively early stage [5]. Flexion contractures of the hip and knee joints are to be expected when the patients become bedridden. As a rule, the patients are able to walk till 25–30 years after the onset of the disease. Often life span is normal and some patients may reach a very advanced age.

Cryptorchidism, hypogenitalism, atrophy of the testes and mental retardation have been described. Cardiac involvement is absent in some families, but in others electrocardiographic abnormalities were a frequent finding [5,7,8].

Polyphasic, short-duration, small-amplitude motor unit potentials are seen during electromyography. Electrophysiologic investigations showed no evidence of motoneuron disfunction [9].

The activity of serum creatine phosphokinase (CPK) is raised, sometimes as high as in Duchenne disease, especially in younger patients [7,11]. It tends to decrease as the disease progresses.

The muscle pathology is also similar to that of Duchenne disease, with foci of necrotic fibres undergoing phagocytosis and basophilic fibres with vesicular nuclei and prominent nucleoli, as well as scattered large, hyaline fibres.

In addition, there is an increase in the number of fibres with internal nuclei. However, type II B fibres, which are rare in Duchenne disease, may be present in the Becker type [3].

Contrary to Duchenne disease, many male patients may have offspring. Consequently, all their daughters are heterozygous and all their sons are unaffected. Therefore, if the daughters have affected sons it would appear that the disease skips a generation. Little information is available concerning the methods of carrier detection. It is possible by estimating the activity of serum CPK, although there is a significant decline with age. Approximately 50 per cent of the known carriers seem to have raised serum CPK activities [4].

The similarity between the Duchenne and the Becker types of muscular dystrophy has led to the conception that these two disorders are merely two extremities of a spectrum of speed of progression. So far, the slowly and the rapidly progressive types have never occurred together in one family, and no intermediary cases have been seen.

It has been postulated that the abnormal genes were allelomorphes and that the two types represented a different mutation of a single gene. There is linkage relationship between the Becker type of X-linked muscular dystrophy and deutan colour blindness. The loci for these two diseases are within measurable distance of each other. Since this is not true for Duchenne disease and colour blindness, it seems that the Duchenne type and the Becker type of muscular dystrophy are not allelic [10].

References **1** Becker,P.E.
Two new families of benign sex-linked recessive muscular dystrophy.
Rev. canad. Biol. 1962, 21 : 551–566

2 Becker,P.E.,Kiener,F.
Eine neue X-chromosomale Muskeldystrophie.
Arch.Psychiat.Nervenkr.1955,193 : 427–448

3 Dubowitz,V.,Brooke,M.H.
Muscle Biopsy: a Modern Approach.
London,Saunders,1973

4 Emery,A.E.H.,Clack,E.R.,Simon,S.,Taylor,J.L.
Detection of carriers of benign X-linked muscular dystrophy.
Brit.med.J.1967,4 : 522–523

5   Emery,A.E.H.,Dreifuss,F.E.
    Unusual type of benign X-linked muscular dystrophy.
    J.Neurol.Neurosurg.Psychiat.1966,29:338–342
6   Kostakow,S.,Derix,F.
    Familienforschung in einer muskeldystrophischen Sippe und
    die Erbprognose ihrer Mitglieder.
    Dtsch.Arch.klin.Med.1937,180:585–606
7   Mabry,C.C.,Roeckel,I.E.,Munich,R.L.,Robertson,D.
    X-linked pseudohypertrophic muscular dystrophy with a late
    onset and slow progression.
    New Engl.J.Med.1965,273:1062–1070
8   Markand,O.N.,North,R.R.,D'Agostino,A.N.,Daly,D.D.
    Benign sex-linked muscular dystrophy. Clinical and
    pathological features.
    Neurology(Minneap.)1969,19:617–633
9   Panayiotopoulos,C.P.,Scarpalezos,S.
    Muscular dystrophies and motoneuron diseases. A
    comparative electrophysiologic study.
    Neurology(Minneap.)1976,26:721–725
10 Skinner,R.,Smith,C.,Emery,A.E.H.
    Linkage between the loci for benign (Becker-type)
    X-borne muscular dystrophy and deutan colour blindness.
    J.med.Genet.1974,11:317–320
11 Zellweger,H.,Hanson,J.W.
    Slowly progressive X-linked recessive muscular dystrophy
    (type IIIb). Report of cases and review of the literature.
    Arch.intern.Med.1967,120:525–535

Facioscapulohumeral (FSH) muscular dystrophy, or Landouzy-Dejerine disease, has an autosomal dominant pattern of inheritance with complete penetrance and markedly variable expressivity.

The age of onset is often very difficult to establish, and varies from 5 to 20 years of age. The initial symptoms may be readily missed by the patient or his doctors, and many patients may remain unaware of their muscular disorder for a long period of time. There is usually very slow progression, with years of apparent arrest, but the rate of progression can be quite variable within the same family. Some patients may have a normal life span with only mild disabilities; others, however, may become severely handicapped after several decades.

The first muscles affected are the muscles of the face — often asymmetric — and of the shoulder girdle. The facial weakness results in inability to wrinkle the forehead, to pucker the lips, to whistle or to close the eyes tightly, so that the eye-lashes often remain visible. The myopathic facies with protrusion of the lips and transverse smile, gives the patient a characteristic appearance, although it is not specific for this type of muscular dystrophy. Some patients may have very slight or even no involvement of the facial musculature, in others facial weakness may be the only sign of the disease.

Loss of ability to raise the arms above the head is a most common initial symptom. Most authors agree that muscular weakness and atrophy is most marked in the sternal head of the pectoralis major, the lattisimus dorsi, the biceps, the triceps and the brachioradialis [6,8,15,17,19]. Notwithstanding the name facioscapulohumeral muscular dystrophy, weakness and wasting of the tibialis anterior muscles is a very striking feature and foot drop may even be an early symptom. In far-advanced stages, severe lordosis and involvement of the pelvic girdle muscles may develop.

Pseudo-hypertrophy and muscular contractures are rarely present. Cardiac involvement is not characteristic of this disease.

Electromyography shows brief, small, abundant motor-unit action potentials. Some electrophysiological investigations suggested a neurogenic influence in FSH muscular dystrophy [2].

The activity of serum creatine phosphokinase (CPK) may be mildly raised, but can be within normal limits. Young patients, with only slight clinical signs usually have a raised CPK level, while after the fifth decade there is a tendency for the CPK activities to drop to normal levels [13].

In the early stages of the disease an increased rate of protein synthesis was observed, but in vitro synthesis of collagen was normal [14].

Muscle pathology includes an increased variability in the size of both fibre types, with many large fibres and sometimes small groups of small angular fibres, reminiscent of denervation atrophy. Occasional necrotic fibres undergoing phagocytosis and basophilic fibres may be present. Groups of small type I moth-eaten or lobulated fibres are frequently seen [4,9]. Cellular infiltrates are common [7,17,20] but it would appear meaningless to treat the patients with corticosteroids because of these inflammatory changes.

Facioscapulohumeral syndrome

Muscular weakness and wasting of facioscapulohumeral distribution may be present in congenital myopathies such as myotubular myopathy [20], central core disease [5] and nemaline myopathy [20]; also in myasthenia gravis [20], polymyositis [3,18], spinal muscular atrophy [1,10,11,16] and in myopathies with abnormal mitochondria, either sporadic [20] or with autosomal dominant inheritance ([12], page 136).

References   1   Acilona,V.,Viruega,A.,Morales,F.,Alberca,R.
Atrofia muscular espinal simulando una distrofia
facioescapulohumeral.
Rev.Neurol.(Barc.)1975,3:363–369
2   Ballantyne,J.P.,Hansen,S.
Computer method for the analysis of evoked motor unit

potentials. 2. Duchenne, limb-girdle, facioscapulohumeral and myotonic muscular dystrophies.
J.Neurol.Neurosurg.Psychiat.1975,38:417–428

3   Bates,D.,Stevens,J.C.,Hudgson,P.
'Polymyositis' with involvement of facial and distal musculature. One form of the facioscapulohumeral syndrome?
J.Neurol.Sci.1973,19:105–108

4   Bethlem,J.,VanWijngaarden,G.K.,DeJong,J.
The incidence of lobulated fibres in the facioscapulohumeral type of muscular dystrophy and the limb-girdle syndrome.
J.neurol.Sci.1973,18:351–358

5   Bethlem,J.,VanWijngaarden,G.K.,Meyer,A.E.F.H.,Fleury,P.
Observations on central core disease
J.Neurol.Sci.1971,14:293–299

6   Bradley,W.G.
Inherited diseases of skeletal muscle.
In:Recent Advances in Clinical Neurology,Vol.1.
W.B.Matthews(ed.).Edinburgh,Livingstone,1955,pp.284–331

7   Brooke,M.H.,Engel,W.K.
The histologic diagnosis of neuromuscular diseases: a review of 79 biopsies.
Arch.phys.Med.1966,47:99–121

8   Chyatte,S.B.,VignosJr,P.J.,Watkins,M.
Early muscular dystrophy: differential patterns of weakness in Duchenne, limb-girdle and facioscapulohumeral types.
Arch.phys.Med.1966,47:499–503

9   Engel,W.K.,Kossmann,R.J.
Selective involvement of histochemical type I muscle fibers in a patient with facioscapulohumeral muscular dystrophy.
Neurology(Minneap.)1963,13:362

10   Fenichel,G.M.,Emery,E.S.,Hunt,P.
Neurogenic atrophy simulating facioscapulohumeral dystrophy. A dominant form.
Arch.Neurol.(Chic.)1967,17:257–260

11   Furukawa,T.,Tsukagoshi,H.,Sugita,H.,Toyokura,Y.
Neurogenic muscular atrophy simulating facioscapulohumeral muscular dystrophy. With particular reference to the heterogeneity of Kugelberg-Welander disease.
J.neurol.Sci.1969,9:389–397

12 Hudgson,P.,Bradley,W.G.,Jenkison,M.
Familial 'mitochondrial' myopathy. A myopathy associated
with disordered oxidative metabolism in muscle fibres.
I. Clinical, electrophysiological and pathological findings.
J.neurol.Sci.1972,16:343–370

13 Hughes,B.P.
Creatine phosphokinase in facioscapulohumeral muscular
dystrophy.
Brit.med.J.1971,3:464–465

14 Ionasescu,V.,Zellweger,H.,Shirk,P.,Conway,T.W.
Abnormal protein synthesis in facioscapulohumeral muscular
dystrophy.
Neurology(Minneap.)1972,22:1286–1292

15 Kazakov,V.M.,Bogorodinsky,D.K.,Znoyko,Z.V.,Skorometz,A.A.
The facio-scapulo-limb (or the facioscapulohumeral) type
of muscular dystrophy.
Europ.Neurol.1974,11:236–260

16 Krüger,H.,Franke,M.
Facioscapulohumerale Form der neurogenen Muskelatrophie.
Psychiat.Neurol.med.Psychol.1974,26:295–301

17 Munsat,T.L.,Piper,D.,Cancilla,P.,Mednick,J.
Inflammatory myopathy with facioscapulohumeral distribution.
Neurology(Minneap.)1972,22:335–347

18 Rothstein,T.L.,Carlson,C.B.,Sumi,S.M.
Polymyositis with facioscapulohumeral distribution.
Arch.Neurol.(Chic.)1971,25:313–319

19 Tyler,F.H.,Stephens,F.E.
Studies in disorders of muscle. II. Clinical manifestations and
inheritance of facioscapulohumeral dystrophy in a large
family.
Ann.intern.Med.1950,32:640–660

20 VanWijngaarden,G.K.,Bethlem,J.
The facioscapulohumeral syndrome.
In:Clinical Studies in Myology.Proceedings of the
2nd International Congress on Muscle Diseases,Perth,
22–26 November 1971.Part 2.B.A.Kakulas(ed.).Amsterdam,
Excerpta Medica,1971,pp.498–501.(Int.Congr.Ser.295)

In scapulo-peroneal myopathy or scapulo-peroneal muscular dystrophy, there is a combination of weakness and wasting of the muscles of the shoulder girdle and of the anterior compartment muscles of the lower limbs. In almost every neuromuscular disease, weakness of these muscles can be found. The only remarkable feature of scapulo-peroneal myopathy is the fact that muscular weakness is mainly confined to these two groups of muscles.

Many authors have described involvement of other muscles as well, for instance the facial muscles, the muscles of the neck or the proximal muscles of both upper and lower limbs. This makes the boundaries of this disorder, and its separation from other neuromuscular diseases, rather vague. In many instances, scapulo-peroneal muscular weakness is merely a certain stage of a slowly progressive condition.

As in every slowly progressive neuromuscular disorder it is often very difficult to state in a patient with scapulo-peroneal muscular involvement, whether this is of neurogenic or myopathic origin. Electromyography is of no great help, because there exists no typical 'myopathic' electromyogram [3]. The histopathological features of a chronic neuropathic condition may resemble those of a myogenic disorder. The histopathological differential diagnosis may be difficult, especially when typical neurogenic features — such as target fibres, large groups of angulated fibres or type grouping — are absent. Moreover, in the scapulo-peroneal syndrome the affected muscles are often very atrophic and therefore not suitable for biopsy, while the clinically non-affected muscles often show very slight and non-specific histological changes.

Therefore, it may sometimes be impossible to determine the site of the primary lesion in a patient with a neuromuscular syndrome of scapulo-peroneal distribution [4].

There are four main groups of diseases presenting this syndrome:

1. Scapulo-peroneal myopathy, in which the primary lesion is thought to be present in the muscle tissue. Sub-groups are sporadic cases [6, 18,20], cases with autosomal dominant [10,19,23] and X-linked recessive inheritance [15,22];

2. Scapulo-peroneal spinal muscular atrophy, in which the primary lesion is present in the anterior horn cells. Sub-groups are sporadic cases [2, 13,16,26], cases with autosomal dominant [8,9,14] and X-linked recessive inheritance [11];

3. Scapulo-peroneal atrophy, in which the primary lesion is present in the peripheral nerves. Sporadic cases without sensory abnormalities have been described [12]. Other sub-groups are sporadic cases [17], and cases with autosomal dominant [1] and autosomal recessive inheritance [24] in which sensory changes were present;

4. Both myopathic and neurogenic lesions were found by some authors in sporadic cases [5] and in cases with autosomal dominant [7], recessive [21] or X-linked recessive inheritance [25].

References 1 Davidenkow,S.
Scapuloperoneal amyotrophy.
Arch.Neurol.Psychiat.(Chic.)1939,41:694–701

2 Emery,E.S.,Fenichel,G.M.,Eng,G.
A spinal muscular atrophy with scapuloperoneal distribution.
Arch.Neurol.(Chic.)1968,18:129–133

3 Engel,W.K.
Brief, small, abundant motor-unit action potentials. A further critique of electromyographic interpretation.
Neurology(Minneap.)1975,25:173–176

4 Feigenbaum,J.A.,Munsat,T.L.
A neuromuscular syndrome of scapuloperoneal distribution.
Bull.Los Angeles neurol.Soc.1970,35:47–57

5 Fotopulos,D.,Schulz,H.
Beitrag zur Pathogenese des scapulo-peronealen Syndroms.
Psychiat.Neurol.med.Psychol.1966,18:129–136

6 Hausmanowa-Petrusewicz,I.,Zielinska,S.
Zur nosologischen Stellung des scapulo-peronealen Syndroms.
Dtsch.Z.Nervenheilk.1962,183:377–382

7 Jennekens,F.G.I.,Busch,H.F.M.,VanHemel,N.M.,
Hoogland,R.A.

Inflammatory myopathy in scapulo-ilio-peroneal atrophy
with cardiopathy.
Brain 1975,98:709–722

8   Kaser,H.E.
Die familiäre scapuloperoneale Muskelatrophie.
Dtsch.Z.Nervenheilk.1964,186:379–394

9   Kaeser,H.E.
Scapuloperoneal muscular atrophy.
Brain 1965,88:407–418

10   Kazakov,V.M.,Bogorodinsky,D.K.,Skorometz,A.A.
Myogenic scapuloperoneal syndrome. Muscular dystrophy
in the K. Kindred. Reexamination of the K. family described
for the first time by Oransky in 1927.
Europ.Neurol.1975,13:350–359

11   Mawatari,S.,Katayama,K.
Scapuloperoneal muscular atrophy with cardiopathy. An
X-linked recessive trait.
Arch.Neurol.(Chic.)1973,28:55–59

12   Meadows,J.C.,Marsden,C.D.
Scapuloperoneal amytrophy.
Arch.Neurol.(Chic.)1969,20:9–12

13   Munsat,T.L.
Infantile scapuloperoneal muscular atrophy.
Neurology(Minneap.)1968,18:285

14   Ricker,K.,Mertens,H.-G.,Schimrigk,K.
The neurogenic scapulo-peroneal syndrome.
Europ.Neurol.1968,1:257–274.

15   Rotthauwe,H.W.,Mortier,W.,Beyer,H.
Neuer Typ einer recessiv X-chromosomal vererbten
Muskeldystrophie: scapulo-humero-distale Muskeldystrophie
mit frühzeitigen Kontrakturen und Herzrhythmusstörungen.
Humangenetik 1972,16:181–200

16   Schuchmann,L.
Spinal muscular atrophy of the scapulo-peroneal type.
Z.Kinderheilk.1970,109:118–123

17   Schwartz,M.S.,Swash,M.
Scapuloperoneal atrophy with sensory involvement:
Davidenkow's syndrome.
J.Neurol.Neurosurg.Psychiat.1975,38:1063–1067

18 Seitz, D.
Zur nosologischen Stellung des sogenannten scapuloperonealen Syndroms.
Dtsch.Z.Nervenheilk.1957,175:547–552

19 Serratrice,G.,Roux,H.,Aquaron,R.,Gambarelli,D.,Baret,J.
Myopathies scapulo-péronières. A propos de 14 observations dont 8 avec atteinte faciale.
Sem.Hôp.Paris 1969,45:2678–2683

20 Steidl,L.,Urbánek,K.
Skapuloperoneální syndrom dystrofického typu.
Cs.Neurol.1973,36:147–150

21 Takahashi,K.,Nakamura,H.,Nakashima,R.
Scapuloperoneal dystrophy associated with neurogenic changes.
J.neurol.Sci.1974,23:575–583

22 Thomas,P.K.,Calne,D.B.,Elliott,C.F.
X-linked scapuloperoneal syndrome.
J.Neurol.Neurosurg.Psychiat.1972,35:208–215

23 Thomas,P.K.,Schott,G.D.,Morgan-Hughes,J.A.
Adult onset scapuloperoneal myopathy.
J.Neurol.Neurosurg.Psychiat.1975,38:1008–1015

24 Tohgi,H.,Tsukagoshi,H.,Toyokura,Y.
Neurogenic scapuloperoneal syndrome with autosomal recessive inheritance.
Clin.Neurol.(Tokyo).1971,11:215–220

25 Waters,D.D.,Nutter,D.O.,Hopkins,L.C.,Dorney,E.R.
Cardiac features of an unusual X-linked humeroperoneal neuromuscular disease.
New Engl.J.Med.1975,293:1017–1022

26 Zellweger,H.,McCormick,W.F.
Scapuloperoneal dystrophy and scapuloperoneal atrophy.
Helv.paediat.Acta 1968,6:643–649

This disease was first described in 1927 by Oransky [3]. One of his families was also reported on in later years [1,2].

Onset is in infancy or in adult life [5]. The involvement of the lower limbs is usually the initial presentation, but in some patients the shoulder girdle muscles are the first to become affected. The disease runs a benign course, with very slow progression. Subsequent involvement of other muscle groups is often seen after several decades. There is a marked variability in the expressivity of the gene. The age at onset, the presenting symptom or sign, the order of the spread of the muscular weakness over the body and the speed of progression, may all vary considerably in different members of the same family.

The weakness and wasting of scapulo-peroneal distribution is often associated with involvement of the facial muscles. Therefore, some authors consider this myopathy as a variant of facioscapulohumeral muscular dystrophy of Landouzy-Dejerine [2,4]. In the latter disease, involvement of the tibialis anterior muscles is frequently present and often an early feature (page 29).

The biceps, triceps and ankle reflexes are usually decreased or absent.

The serum CPK activity may be normal or slightly raised.

The electromyogram shows small-amplitude, excessively abundant and polyphasic action potentials. Motor nerve conduction velocities are normal.

Muscle biopsy shows marked variation in the diameter of both type I and type II fibres, increase in the number of fibres with internal nuclei, and moth-eaten or lobulated type I fibres. In the end stages a marked increase of fat and connective tissue may be seen.

References   1   Davidenkow,S.
                 Scapuloperoneal amyotrophy.
                 Arch.Neurol.Psychiat.(Chic.)1939,41:694–701
             2   Kazakov,V.M.,Bogorodinsky,D.K.,Skorometz,A.A.
                 Myogenic scapuloperoneal syndrome. Muscular dystrophy

in the K. Kindred. Reexamination of the K. family described for the first time by Oransky in 1927.
Europ.Neurol.1975,13:350–359

3 Oransky,W.
Ueber einen hereditären Typus progressiver Muskeldystrophie.
Dtsch.Z.Nervenheilk.1927,99:147–155

4 Serratrice,G.,Roux,H.,Aquaron,R.,Gambarelli,D.,Baret,J.
Myopathies scapulo-péronières. A propos de 14 observations dont 8 avec atteinte faciale.
Sem.Hôp.Paris 1969,45:2678–2683

5 Thomas,P.K.,Schott,G.D.,Morgan-Hughes,J.A.
Adult onset scapuloperoneal myopathy.
J.Neurol.Neurosurg.Psychiat.1975,38:1008–1015

In 1972, Rotthauwe, Mortier and Beyer [2] described an X-linked disease which they named scapulo-humero-distal muscular dystrophy. In three generations of a German pedigree, 17 males were affected.

The first manifestation of the disease developed within the first decade and consisted of muscular contractures without muscular weakness. In the early stage contractures of the gastrocnemius muscles were present, followed by shortening of the muscles of the neck, the paravertebral musculature, the biceps brachii muscles and the hamstrings. Most patients were unable to bend forward normally, while the movements of the head were also markedly restricted.

In the second decade muscular weakness developed, mainly involving the deltoids and pectoralis muscles, the muscles of the upper arms, the extensors of the hands, fingers and feet. Five patients also showed weakness of the facial musculature. The other muscles of the shoulder girdle and the musculature of the pelvic girdle were relatively spared, even in very advanced cases. Marked atrophy — especially of the muscles of the upper arms, the lower legs and the cheeks — and areflexia were often present.

In five patients there was cardiopathy with a partial or complete atrioventricular block.

Elevation of the serum creatine phosphokinase activity was found in six young patients.

Electromyography showed motor unit potentials of brief duration and small amplitude, as well as fibrillation potentials. Motor and sensory nerve conduction velocities were normal.

Muscle biopsy showed variation in fibre diameter, increase of internal nuclei, occasional necrotic fibres, increase of endomysial connective tissue, and round-cell infiltrates. In one biopsy, there was type I fibre predominance.

The mean age at death was 45 years; all patients died suddenly, presumably due to cardiac arrest.

On examination, the definite carriers did not show any features of a neuromuscular disease, while the serum CPK activity was normal. One heterozygote showed a partial atrioventricular block.

Also in 1972, Thomas, Calne and Elliott [3] reported on an X-linked scapulo-peroneal syndrome. The age at onset was about 5 years, with slow
progression. Pes cavus and contractures of the elbows were present
in most patients, while limitation of neck flexion was found in one case.
The electromyographic findings were equivocal. Serum CPK activity was
increased. Autopsy of one patient showed the muscle histopathology to be
in favour of a myopathy. The sciatic nerve was normal. The spinal cord was
not examined and no histochemistry of the muscle tissue was carried out.
Cardiomyopathy was a feature in three patients, and probably the cause
of death in one patient. The disease was linked with deutan colour blindness.

An X-linked scapulo-peroneal muscular atrophy in a Japanese family was
described in 1973 by Mawatari and Katayama [1]. The age at onset was
between 7 and 10 years. The initial symptom was shortness of the Achilles
tendons. Scapulo-peroneal weakness and atrophy was associated with
limitation of flexion of the neck. In one patient fasciculations were
present.
The electromyogram showed neurogenic features; motor nerve conduction
velocities were normal, suggesting a primary lesion of the anterior horn
cells.
In one case a biopsy was performed in which groups of small fibres were
seen, compatible with a neurogenic lesion.
In addition, a cardiopathy with conduction defects was found in the
patients and the female carriers.

In 1975, Waters, Nutter, Hopkins and Dorney [4] described an X-linked
disorder that they called humeroperoneal neuromuscular disease. They
reported on two American families in which respectively 16 and 21 males
were affected.
The initial manifestation of the disease was muscular weakness in the
upper arms between the ages of 2 and 10 years. Slowly progressive involvement of proximal arm muscles and distal leg muscles stabilized at

approximately 20 years of age. Shortening of Achilles tendons, elbow contractures and marked restriction of neck flexion, were characteristic of the clinical picture.

The serum CPK activity was increased. Electromyographic and histopathological investigations revealed abnormalities that were considered to be consistent with both neurogenic and primary myopathic involvement. Electrocardiography showed a spectrum of atrial rhythm and conduction disturbances that ranged from abnormal waves to permanent atrial paralysis in four patients.

Fifteen of the 37 patients died suddenly before the age of 50 years.

The authors thought that this disease was similar to scapulo-humero-distal muscular dystrophy [2].

References   1   Mawatari,S.,Katayama,K.
                       Scapuloperoneal muscular atrophy with cardiopathy.
                       An X-linked recessive trait.
                       Arch.Neurol.(Chic.)1973,28:55–59
                 2   Rotthauwe,H.W.,Mortier,W.,Beyer,H.
                       Neuer Typ einer recessiv X-chromosomal vererbten
                       Muskeldystrophie: scapulo-humero-distale Muskeldystrophie
                       mit frühzeitigen Kontrakturen und Herzrhythmusstörungen.
                       Humangenetik 1972,16:181–200
                 3   Thomas,P.K.,Calne,D.B.,Elliott,C.F.
                       X-linked scapuloperoneal syndrome.
                       J.Neurol.Neurosurg.Psychiat.1972,35:208–215
                 4   Waters,D.D.,Nutter,D.O.,Hopkins,L.C.,Dorney,E.R.
                       Cardiac features of an unusual X-linked humeroperoneal
                       neuromuscular disease.
                       New Engl.J.Med.1975,293:1017–1022

Some patients may suffer from a progressive condition in which weakness and atrophy of the muscles of the shoulder and pelvic girdles and of the proximal limbs, develop.

Although these patients are often considered to be suffering from limb-girdle muscular dystrophy, it is doubtful if all the cases described were of a similar nature and if this condition is in fact a real entity. Most cases were sporadic or had an autosomal recessive mode of inheritance [1,2].

There is a wide variation in the age of onset, the initial sign or symptom, the spread of the muscular weakness over the body, the speed of progression, the serum creatine phosphokinase activities and the histopathological picture. Because of this heterogeneity, the name limb-girdle syndrome is preferred. Many myopathies may present this syndrome in a certain phase of development.

References   **1**   Becker,P.E.
Dystrophia musculorum progressiva. Eine genetische und klinische Untersuchung der Muskeldystrophien. Stuttgart,Thieme,1953.(Sammlung psychiatrischer und neurologischer Einzeldarstellungen)

  2   Jackson,C.E.,Strehler,D.A.
Limb-girdle muscular dystrophy: clinical manifestations and detection of preclinical disease.
Pediatrics 1968,41:495 502

In 1976, Bethlem and Van Wijngaarden [1] described 3 families in The Netherlands in which 28 members suffered from a benign myopathy. Although the motor development was normal, all patients observed some muscular symptoms around the fifth year of life. They could not run, tended to fall down easily, had difficulty with jumping and skipping and were very poor at gymnastics. After these early manifestations of the disease, the progression was very slow. Sometimes the muscular weakness worsened after pregnancy or in middle age. Nevertheless, most adult patients succeeded in earning their living, had a normal family life, and maintained a good social level. Life expectancy was not shortened by the disease and many patients reached old age (seventh and eighth decades).

On examination the patients presented a generalized moderate muscular weakness and atrophy, without involvement of the cranial muscles. Weakness of the flexors of the head was present in almost all patients. Proximal muscles were more involved than the distal, the extensors more than the flexors. A frequent finding was flexion contractures of the elbows and of the interphalangeal joints of the last four fingers (attributed to a more severe paresis of the extensor digitorum communis muscle) and plantar flexion contracture of the ankles.

Congenital torticollis due to unilateral shortening of a sternocleidomastoid muscle was present in 4 out of 28 patients. The reflexes were hypoactive or absent and this did not always correlate with the severity of the muscular weakness.

The serum creatine phosphokinase activity was usually normal or slightly increased.

Electromyographic investigations were equivocal, the motor nerve conduction velocities were normal.

Muscle biopsies revealed large and small fibres of both types, without specific structural changes. Lobulated type I fibres were found in half the cases. There was a moderate increase in the number of fibres with internal nuclei. A marked increase of fatty tissue and almost no increase of connective tissue were observed in the later stages.

Electron microscopy revealed no specific changes.

Post-mortem examination in one case, including motor neuron cell counts of the lumbosacral cord, did not show convincing features of a neurogenic disorder.

In all pedigrees, the disease was transmitted as an autosomal dominant trait.

Reference   **1**   Bethlem,J.,VanWijngaarden,G.K.
Benign myopathy, with autosomal dominant inheritance.
Brain 1976,99:91–100

In 1967, Henson, Muller and DeMyer [1] reported on a family with a limb-girdle syndrome in which the affected members through two generations were all females.

The young girls showed pathologic lumbar lordosis and slight weakness of the muscles of the shoulder and pelvic girdles.

The adult females had marked weakness and wasting of the limb-girdle muscles and excessive lumbar lordosis. The deep tendon reflexes were absent. The activity of the serum creatine phosphokinase was mildly raised. Electromyography showed polyphasic and brief-duration, low-amplitude motor unit potentials.

Muscle pathology revealed considerable variation in muscle size, with many small and hypertrophied fibres. Necrotic fibres, undergoing phagocytosis, and basophilic fibres with vesicular nuclei were present. A clearcut mosaic of type I and type II fibres could not be recognized in sections stained for oxidative enzyme activities.

According to the authors the limitation of the disease to females can be best explained by an autosomal mode of inheritance with the expression limited to females.

Reference 1 Henson,T.E.,Muller,J.,DeMyer,W.E.
Hereditary myopathy limited to females.
Arch.Neurol.(Chic.)1967,17:238–247

In 1967, Stanton and Strong [1] described a 21-year-old woman who, during the last $3\frac{1}{2}$ years, had a progressive weakness of both limb-girdles without local wasting. The pelvic girdle musculature was more involved than the shoulder girdle. The neck and trunk muscles were also paretic. The tendon reflexes were all moderately diminished.

Laboratory findings, including activity of serum creatine phosphokinase, were within normal limits.

Muscle pathology consisted of considerable variation in fibre size, some increase of sarcolemmal nuclei and occasional central nuclei.

The muscular weakness did not respond to corticosteroid therapy. During two pregnancies there was a marked improvement of the muscular weakness that deteriorated again after delivery.

In view of the spontaneous improvement which had occurred in the pregnancies, the patient was given massive doses of oestrogen and progestogen. During this treatment — already continued for 6 years when the paper was published — her condition remained remarkably good, although she had some difficulty climbing stairs or on to a bus.

Reference   1   Stanton,J.B.,Strong,J.A.
Myopathy remitting in pregnancy and responding to high-dosage oestrogen and progestogen therapy.
Lancet 1967,II:275–277

In some patients there may be weakness limited to the quadriceps femoris muscles, with very slow or no progression.

In some patients the paresis and atrophy was mainly confined to the distal portion of the quadriceps muscles [1,3–5] or to the vastus medialis muscles [2,6].

In a few cases, clinical [4] or electromyographical [5] evidence of a more generalized myopathy was observed.

The patellar reflexes were hypoactive or absent. The serum creatine phosphokinase activity may be mildly raised. Electromyography showed brief-duration, small-amplitude and polyphasic motor unit potentials in most cases.

Muscle biopsy studies revealed small and large fibres, necrotic fibres undergoing phagocytosis, vacuolation, basophilic fibres with vesicular nuclei and prominent nucleoli, ringed fibres and an increase in the number of fibres with internal nuclei. Marked proliferation of connective and fat tissue was seen in most biopsies. A normal distribution of type I and type II fibres was observed in 2 cases [5]. Numerous inflammatory cells, mostly lymphocytes and plasma cells, were present in one case [4].

Familial occurrence (2 brothers) has been described [5], but all other observations were of isolated cases.

The nosology of this syndrome remains obscure. It has been considered as a chronic polymyositis by some authors, and as a peculiar kind of muscular dystrophy by others.

References   1   Bramwell, E.
Observations on myopathy.
Proc.roy.Soc.Med.(Sect.Neurol.)1922,16:1–12
2   Denny-Brown, D.
Myopathic weakness of quadriceps.
Proc.roy.Soc.Med.1939,32:867–869
3   Mumenthaler, M., Bosch, T., Katzenstein, E., Lehner, F.
Ueber den isolierten Befall des M. quadriceps femoris bei der Dystrophia musculorum progressiva.
Confin.neurol.1958,18:416–441

4 Turner,J.W.A.,Heathfield,K.W.G.
Quadriceps myopathy occurring in middle age.
J.Neurol.Neurosurg.Psychiat.1961,24:18–21
5 VanWijngaarden,G.K.,Hagen,C.J.,Bethlem,J.,Meyer,A.E.F.H.
Myopathy of the quadriceps muscles.
J.neurol.Sci.1968,7:201–206
6 Walton,J.N.
Two cases of myopathy limited to the quadriceps.
J.Neurol.Neurosurg.Psychiat.1956,19:106–108

Although a disease of the lower motor neuron and not a myopathy, this disorder will be mentioned here in brief because it has often been mis-diagnosed as limb-girdle muscular dystrophy.

It is also named Wohlfart-Kugelberg-Welander disease, and is considered to be a disorder with an autosomal recessive mode of inheritance, although many sporadic cases have been described [1,3,4].

Onset varies from birth to the fifth decade. Reduced fetal movements and floppiness at birth are often the initial features, but for many parents, or patients, it is difficult to state the exact age of the first manifestations, mainly because of the insidious onset of the disease.

The disorder is usually slowly progressive. The grade of disability does not correlate to the patients' age, the age at onset or the duration of the disease.

The muscles of the pelvic girdle and proximal leg muscles are usually first and more severely involved than the muscles of the upper part of the body. In more advanced cases the muscles of the neck and the distal muscles of the extremities are also affected. In a number of patients weakness of the muscles innervated by the cranial nerves (facial muscles, tongue, pharynx and extra-ocular muscles) is observed. In some patients hyper-trophy of the calf muscles may be present.

Fasciculations are seen in about half the cases, sometimes limited to the tongue.

The deep tendon reflexes are hypoactive or absent, but occasionally there may be extensor plantar reflexes and other evidences of upper motor neuron involvement. The activity of serum creatine phosphokinase is usually normal in infants and tends to be raised around puberty [2,4].

Electromyographic findings include spontaneous activity, reduced full effort pattern, increased potential amplitude and duration, and increased motor unit territory [1]. Muscle biopsy investigation reveals the features of a chronic denervation, including fibre type grouping or target fibres.

References 1 Emery,A.E.H.,Hausmanowa-Petrusewicz,I.,Davie,A.M.,
Holloway,S.,Skinner,R.,Borkowska,J.
International collaborative study of the spinal muscular
atrophies. Part 1. Analysis of clinical and laboratory data.
J.neurol.Sci.1976,29:83–94

2 Heyck,H.,Laudahn,G.
Muscle and Serum Enzymes in Muscular Dystrophy and
Neurogenic Muscular Atrophy. A comparative study.
Amsterdam,Excerpta Medica,1967,pp.232–240.
(Int.Congr.Ser.147).

3 Namba,T.,Aberfeld,D.C.,Grob,D.
Chronic proximal spinal muscular atrophy.
J.neurol.Sci.1970,11:401–423

4 VanWijngaarden,G.K.,Bethlem,J.
Benign infantile spinal muscular atrophy. A prospective study.
Brain 1973,96:163–170

Most distal myopathies so far described, are rare autosomal dominantly inherited diseases, in which the initial muscular weakness is present either
in the feet or in the hands, with no, or only slow, progression.

In many of the reports, examinations were incomplete, according to
modern concepts, leaving the possibility that in some instances a neurogenic pathogenesis cannot be ruled out with certainty.

In general, it has often appeared to be wrong to classify diseases according
to the age at onset. However, at present there is no other way than to
subdivide the distal myopathies into congenital, infantile and late onset
types.

A congenital distal myopathy was first described in 1968 by Heyck, Lüders and Wolter [1] in a 32-year-old woman. The initial weakness was present in the extensors of the feet. After 29 years, weakness of the extensors of the hands and fingers developed. The tendon reflexes of the lower extremities were absent. The myopathic nature of this non-familial condition was based on electromyography and conventional histopathological studies of three muscle biopsies.

A dominant mode of transmission was found in a family in which three males were suffering from a non-progressive, congenital distal myopathy [2]. Muscular weakness was limited to the legs. There was no wasting of the involved muscles, but marked hypertrophy of the calf muscles was present. The reflexes were low or absent. No motor nerve conduction velocities were mentioned. Muscle biopsy in one case showed type I fibre predominance, variation in fibre diameter and increase in the number of fibres with internal nuclei. In about 10–20 per cent of the type I fibres large collections of mitochondria, abnormal in shape and structure, were present.

References   **1**   Heyck,H.,Lüders,C.J.,Wolter,M.
Ueber eine kongenitale distale Muskeldystrophie mit
benigner Progredienz.
Nervenarzt 1968,39:549–552

2   Lapresle,J.,Fardeau,M.,Godet-Guillain,J.
Myopathie distale et congénitale, avec hypertrophie des
mollets. Présence d'anomalies mitochondriales à
la biopsie musculaire.
J.neurol.Sci.1972,17:87–102

The first description of a distal myopathy with onset in infancy has been given by Magee and De Jong [2]. The onset of this autosomal dominantly inherited disease was evident at the age of 2 years, but probably the disorder was already present at birth.

The initial sign consisted of bilateral foot drop. Weakness of the hands and forearms became evident during childhood, with a predilection for the extensors of the fingers. After the age of 18 years there was no obvious progression.

In one patient, the myopathic nature of the disorder was based on electromyographic findings and conventional histological studies of three biopsies, including the right vastus lateralis muscle that also clinically appeared to be mildly paretic.

Similar cases were described in another paper [4], but later studies showed target fibres in a muscle biopsy [1] and therefore these patients were considered to be suffering from a chronic neurogenic condition.

Another, also probably autosomal dominantly inherited distal myopathy — with weakness confined to the distal muscles of the legs at the age of 5 years — was associated with hyperglycaemia and hyperketonaemia [3]. The latter did not seem to be a simple consequence of the patient's diabetes. High levels of plasma free fatty acids and raised serum CPK activity were also present.

Muscle biopsy revealed accumulations of abnormal mitochondria and of lipid, while some fibres also contained large subsarcolemmal collections of glycogen.

The paternal grandfather, father and twin brother of the female proband were clinically unaffected; however, increased serum CPK activity and hyperglycaemia were observed.

References   1   Bethlem,J.
                     Unpublished observations.
               2   Magee,K.R.,DeJong,R.N.
                     Hereditary distal myopathy with onset in infancy.
                     Arch.Neurol.(Chic.)1965,13:387–390

3 Salmon,M.A.,Esiri,M.M.,Ruderman,N.B.
Myopathic disorder associated with mitochondrial
abnormalities, hyperglycaemia, and hyperketonaemia.
Lancet 1971,II:290–293

4 VanderDoesdeWillebois,A.E.M.,Bethlem,J.,Meyer,A.E.F.H.,
Simons,A.J.R.
Distal myopathy with onset in early infancy.
Neurology(Minneap.)1968,18:383–390

Myopathia distalis tarda hereditaria or Welander disease is an autosomal dominantly inherited late onset distal myopathy with a predominance in males. It was first described by Welander [7] in 249 patients belonging to 72 Swedish pedigrees. The age of onset was around 50 years, onset before the age of 40 years was very uncommon. The first complaints consisted of coldness of the hands and clumsiness in performing fine movements with the fingers, such as fastening buttons or picking up small objects. This was followed by weakness and wasting of the extensors and small muscles of the hands, and subsequent involvement of the feet. The symptoms often started unilaterally in the thumb and/or index finger. Occasionally, the first signs were observed in the feet or simultaneously in both hands and feet. Even after 25 years the muscular features remained confined to the distal extensor muscles of the upper and lower limbs. It was very uncommon to find proximal weakness or involvement of the distal flexor muscles. In cases of long duration, the ankle reflexes were absent, but otherwise the reflexes were normal. The disease ran a slow progressive course and had no influence on life expectancy.

The electromyogram showed brief-duration and small-amplitude motor unit potentials with increased polyphasic forms.

In the muscle biopsies a marked variation in fibre size was seen with an increase in the number of fibres with internal nuclei and proliferation of connective tissue. Vacuoles were also present in some biopsies. Examination of the spinal cord, nerve roots and peripheral nerves in three autopsy cases revealed no abnormalities.

In later years other authors found indications of a neurogenic factor in the pathogenesis of Welander disease. In another study from Sweden [1] histochemical investigation of 13 muscle biopsies showed selective atrophy of type I fibres, with a bimodal size distribution. In more advanced stages, marked changes in myofibrillar ATPase staining characteristics were seen, and differentiation of type I and type II fibres was not possible.

Electron microscopy in one case showed absence of nerve terminals from the post-synaptic regions [2]. Pathological involvement of the terminal nerve twigs or the motor end-plates was also suggested by electrophysiological studies in 6 patients [5].

Late onset distal myopathy with gradual onset of weakness and atrophy in the distal muscles of the lower limbs, and subsequent involvement of the distal muscles of the upper extremities and proximal limb muscles, has also been described [4]. Cardiomyopathy was present in one case. The disease was probably of autosomal dominant inheritance. In general, the patients showed more severe and widespread progressive weakness than in Welander disease.

Muscle histopathology revealed no selective fibre type atrophy or type grouping; a consistent finding was the presence of vacuoles in the muscle fibres.

In one case there was slightly diminished vibratory sense in the toes and minimally decreased perception of superficial pain below the ankles. Autopsy revealed mild degenerative changes in peripheral nerves and spinal roots. These findings were thought to be superimposed on the primary muscle disease.

Late onset muscular dystrophy, with involvement of the flexors as well as extensors of forearms and lower legs and of the intrinsic muscles of hands and feet, was found in 2 brothers [6]. Onset was at 15 and 22 years. Three affected sisters had a later onset (35–50 years), and showed weakness of the extensors of the forearms and the intrinsic muscles of the hands. However, the legs were not examined because no permission for complete examination was obtained.

In one patient muscle pathology of paraffin sections was equivocal. Results of the intravital methylene blue staining technic were comparable to those found in moderately advanced muscular dystrophy.

In rare instances, late onset distal muscular weakness may be the presenting symptom of polymyositis [3] or it may be observed in ocular myopathy (page 60).

References   1   Edström,L.
Histochemical and histopathological changes in skeletal
muscle in late-onset hereditary distal myopathy (Welander).
J.neurol.Sci.1975,26:147–157

2   Engel,A.G.,Jerusalem,F.,Tsujihata,M.,Gomez,M.R.
The neuromuscular junction in myopathies. A quantitative
ultrastructural study.
In:Recent Advances in Myology.Proceedings of the 3rd
international congress on muscle diseases,Newcastle
upon Tyne,15–21 September,1974.W.G.Bradley,D.Gardner-
Medwin,J.N.Walton(eds.).Amsterdam,Excerpta Medica,
1974,pp.132–143.(Int.Congr.Ser.360).

3   Hollinrake,K.
Polymyositis presenting as distal muscle weakness.
A case report.
J.neurol.Sci.1969,8:479–484

4   Markesbery,W.R.,Griggs,R.C.,Leach,R.P.,Lapham,L.W.
Late onset hereditary distal myopathy.
Neurology(Minneap.)1974,24:127–134

5   Stålberg,E.,Ekstedt,J.
Signs of neuropathy in distal hereditary myopathy (Welander).
Electroenceph.clin.Neurophysiol.1969,29:343

6   Sumner,D.,Crawfurd,M.d'A.,Harriman,D.G.F.
Distal muscular dystrophy in an English family.
Brain 1971,94:51–60

7   Welander,L.
Myopathia distalis tarda hereditaria. 249 Examined cases
in 72 pedigrees.
Acta med.scand.1951,Suppl.265,141:1–124

Chronic progressive external ophthalmoplegia was first described by Von Gräfe (1868). It was considered to be of nuclear origin subsequent to the publication by Möbius (1900). Although some authors suggested that the disorder was myopathic and not due to a primary involvement of the oculomotor cells in the brain stem, this concept was only generally accepted following the study by Kiloh and Nevin (1951).

In normal eye muscles a marked variation in fibre diameter, many internal nuclei, sarcoplasmic masses and ringed fibres, and a large amount of endomysial connective tissue may be present. These findings together with the complicated normal histochemical features [2] make the interpretation of the histopathological findings in a biopsy from an extraocular muscle very difficult.

The same holds true for the interpretation of the electromyographic findings in ocular muscles. The motor units in the ocular muscles contain very few muscle fibres (approximately 10–20 fibres). The mean duration of normal extraocular muscle motor unit potentials is very short (1–2 msec). The firing rate is much faster than that of the limb muscles. This makes it difficult to detect a reduction in the fibre content of the motor units. The short normal motor unit potentials may be very difficult to distinguish from abnormal action potentials in ocular neuromuscular disorders.

Unless there are marked neurogenic changes, the diagnostic value of ocular electromyography in progressive external ophthalmoplegia is limited and uncertain.

There are many syndromes in which progressive external ophthalmoplegia is the outstanding, and very often the first, clinical symptom [1,3].

The classification of these disorders is extremely difficult and remains arbitrary, especially because the genetic aspects, the clinical picture, the laboratory findings and the pathology vary from case to case. Moreover, in most cases no metabolic defect could be established.

Clinical diagnosis is complicated by the fact that the progression of the disorder may be very slow and gradual, so that it can take many years before another symptom develops. Therefore, the findings during the first examination often present an incomplete clinical picture, and this may constitute an additional factor to the confusion in the literature about the ocular myopathies. Even in patients in which there is a familial occurrence of the disease there may be a marked difference in clinical expression.

From the practical point of view, it seems justified to recognize the following three syndromes: ocular myopathy (page 60), oculopharyngeal myopathy (page 61) and oculocraniosomatic neuromuscular disease (page 63).

References   1   Drachman,D.A.
                      Ophthalmoplegia plus; a classification of the disorders
                      associated with progressive external ophthalmoplegia.
                      In:Handbook of Clinical Neurology.P.J.Vinken,G.W.Bruyn
                      (eds.).Vol.22,part2:System disorders and atrophies.
                      Amsterdam,North-Holland,1975,pp.203–216
                 2   Durston,J.H.J.
                      Histochemistry of primate extraocular muscles and the
                      changes of denervation.
                      Brit.J.Ophthal.1974,58:193–216
                 3   Rowland,L.P.
                      Progressive external ophthalmoplegia.
                      In:Handbook of Clinical Neurology.P.J.Vinken,G.W.Bruyn
                      (eds.).Vol.22,part2:System disorders and atrophies.
                      Amsterdam,North-Holland,1975,pp.177–202

In this slowly progressive condition the first symptom is ptosis, usually bilateral and starting at any time, from infancy to old age. The patient has the tendency to tilt his head backwards and to wrinkle his forehead in order to compensate for the weakness of the levator muscles. Drooping of the eyelids is followed by weakness of the other extra-ocular muscles. The constrictor muscles of the iris are spared and hence the pupils and pupillary reactions remain normal. The involvement of the extraocular muscles occurs so insidiously and the progression is so slow that the patient generally does not complain of diplopia.

After many years there may be subsequent spread to the facial muscles, the muscles of the neck and of the limbs, especially of the upper arms ('descending ocular myopathy'). The upper facial muscles are usually weaker than the lower [1]. In rare cases there is predominance of weakness and atrophy of the distal muscles of the extremities [2,3].

The activity of serum creatine phosphokinase may be moderately increased even in patients in whom there is no weakness of the muscles of the extremities.

In about half the cases the disorder is inherited, either as a recessive or a dominant trait.

References 1 Danta,G.,Hilton,R.C.,Lynch,P.G.
               Chronic progressive external ophthalmoplegia.
               Brain 1975,98:473–492
            2 Satoyoshi,E.,Murakami,K.,Kowa,H.,Kinoshita,M.,Torii,J.
               Distal involvement of the extremities in ocular myopathy.
               Amer.J.Ophthal.1965,59:668–673
            3 Schotland,D.L.,Rowland,L.P.
               Muscular dystrophy. Features of ocular myopathy, distal
               myopathy, and myotonic dystrophy.
               Arch.Neurol.(Chic.)1964,10:433–445

Oculopharyngeal myopathy has also been named oculopharyngeal muscular dystrophy, hereditary late onset ptosis and dysphagia, ocular myopathy with dysphagia and progressive muscular dystrophy with ptosis and dysphagia.

The first publication of oculopharyngeal myopathy was given by Taylor as early as 1915. He described a French-Canadian family in which the siblings suffered from ptosis and dysphagia. The onset of the disease was approximately at the age of 50 years. Since then other studies have been published [1–4,7,9,10], most of them concerning patients of French-Canadian descent [1,2,4,7,9]. In fact it was shown that all reported cases of French-Canadian stock could be traced to one single common ancestor who landed in Quebec from France in 1634.

This myopathy is usually restricted to the cranial muscles, and is characterized by slowly progressive ocular ptosis and dysphagia. In addition there may be slight involvement of the orbicularis oris, orbicularis oculi, temporalis, masseter and limb muscles. It is noteworthy, however, that most patients do not develop weakness of any of the other extra-ocular muscles.

Muscle biopsy showed marked variation in fibre size, scattered small angulated fibres and rimmed vacuoles from which fine filaments arose [5]. These vacuoles were usually present in the type I fibres. In the trichrome stained sections the vacuoles were surrounded by a rim of red staining material.

Electron microscopy revealed collections of abnormally large and bizarrely structured mitochondria and 'fingerprint' inclusions [8].

Although sporadic and autosomal recessive [6] cases occur, an autosomal dominant mode of inheritance was found in most familial cases.

References   1   Amyot,R.
Hereditary, familial and acquired ptosis of late onset.
Canad.med.Ass.J.1948,59:434

2   Barbeau,A.
    The syndrome of hereditary late onset ptosis and dysphagia
    in French Canada.
    In:Symposium über progressive Muskeldystrophie.
    E.Kühn(ed.).Berlin,Springer,1966,pp.102–109
3   Campanella,G.,Filla,A.,Serlenga,L.,Federico,A.,Buscaino,G.A.
    Myopathie oculo-pharyngée. Observations histochimiques
    musculaires et dosage des immunoglobulines du sérum
    dans une famille italienne.
    Rev.Neurol.1975,131:615–628
4   Bray,G.M.,Kaarsoo,M.,Ross,R.T.
    Ocular myopathy with dysphagia.
    Neurology(Minneap.)1965,15:678–684
5   Dubowitz,V.,Brooke,M.H.
    Muscle Biopsy: a modern approach.
    London,Saunders,1973
6   Fried,K.,Arlozorov,A.,Spira,R.
    Autosomal recessive oculopharyngeal muscular dystrophy.
    J.med.Genet.1975,12:416–418
7   Hayes,R.,London,W.,Seidman,J.,Embree,L.
    Oculopharyngeal muscular dystrophy.
    New Engl.J.Med.1963,268:163
8   Julien,J.,Vital,C.,Vallat,J.M.,Vallat,M.,LeBlanc,M.
    Oculopharyngeal muscular dystrophy. A case with abnormal
    mitochondria and 'fingerprint' inclusions.
    J.neurol.Sci.1974,21:165–169
9   Peterman,A.F.,Lillington,G.A.,Jamplis,R.W.
    Progressive muscular dystrophy with ptosis and dysphagia.
    Arch.Neurol.(Chic.)1964,10:38–41
10 Victor,M.,Hayes,R.,Adams,R.D.
    Oculopharyngeal muscular dystrophy. A familial disease
    of late life characterized by dysphagia and progressive ptosis
    of the eyelids.
    New Engl.J.Med.1962,267:1267–1272

Progressive external ophthalmoplegia may be found in association with a variety of neurological and other abnormalities. In 1958 Kearns and Sayre [6] reported on two patients who showed the triad external ophthalmoplegia, retinitis pigmentosa and complete heart block. In addition other features were described: weakness of facial, pharyngeal, trunk and extremity muscles, neural deafness, small stature, electroencephalographic changes, marked increase in cerebrospinal fluid protein [5], peripheral neuropathy, cerebellar ataxia [12], optic atrophy [1], endocrine disturbances and dementia.

Many names were given to these syndromes, for instance ophthalmoplegia plus [1], Kearns-Shy syndrome [4], oculoskeletal myopathy [8], oculocranioskeletal neuromuscular disease [13].

Olson, Engel, Walsh and Einaugler [10] were the first to draw attention to the presence of 'ragged-red fibres' (page 125) in the clinically normal or only minimally weak limb muscles. These fibres show an abnormal amount of lipid droplets and contain clusters of normal and abnormal mitochondria in which paracrystalline inclusions may be present. The authors found that these abnormal fibres were nearly always of type I.

The number of abnormal fibres ranged from 1 to 5 per cent.

Other authors [8] found both fibre types affected, their number ranging from 8 to 18 per cent. There appeared to be no correlation between the number of abnormal fibres and the severity of the muscle weakness or the duration of the symptoms.

Similar mitochondrial abnormalities were found in the extra-ocular muscles [14].

Although there are indications that both myopathic and neuropathic factors are present in the disease, no abnormalities were found in the motor endplates of a skeletal muscle biopsy, while the terminal innervation ratio was normal [2]. Involvement of the central nervous system is indicated by many clinical findings, such as cerebellar ataxia, dementia, electroencephalographic abnormalities and the elevated cerebrospinal fluid protein.

Various neuropathological findings in the brain, including widespread spongiform changes, were found and appeared to be non-specific.

Mitochondrial abnormalittes were shown by electron microscopy in the neuropil of the cerebellum [11]. Abnormal mitochondria were also seen in the liver [3,9] and in more than half of the secretory cells of the eccrine sweat glands in the skin [4].

Although virtually all the described patients were isolated cases, the observation of familial occurrence of the disease [13] suggests an auto-somal recessive pattern of inheritance.

It is interesting that ragged-red type I fibres were also found in a patient with generalized muscle weakness, mental retardation, short stature, epilepsy, chorioretinitis, deafness, ataxia, abnormalities of the electro-encephalogram and electrocardiogram, elevated cerebrospinal fluid protein and abnormal carbohydrate metabolism, but without any symptoms of external ophthalmoplegia [7].

This case demonstrates the wide spectrum of signs, beginning with those which are merely restricted to the extraocular muscles, followed by the many manifestations of oculocraniosomatic neuromuscular disease, and finally the same disorder without involvement of the ocular muscles.

References 1 Drachman,D.A.
Ophthalmoplegia plus. The neurodegenerative disorders associated with progressive external ophthalmoplegia.
Arch.Neurol.(Chic.)1968,18:654–674

2 Gérard,J.M.,Rétif,J.,Telerman-Toppet,N.,Demols,E.,Coërs,C.
Myopathie mitochondriale associée à une ophthalmoplégie externe progressive.
Acta neurol.belg.1974,74:284–296

3 Gonatas,N.K.,Evangelista,I.,andMartin,J.
A generalized disorder of nervous system, skeletal muscle and heart resembling Refsum's disease and Hurler's syndrome.
II. Ultrastructure.
Amer.J.Med.1967,42:169–178

4   Karpati,G.,Carpenter,S.,Larbrisseau,A.,Lafontaine,R.
     The Kearns-Shy syndrome. A multisystem disease with
     mitochondrial abnormality demonstrated in skeletal muscle
     and skin.
     J.neurol.Sci.1973,19:133–151
5   Kearns,T.P.
     External ophthalmoplegia, pigmentary degeneration of
     the retina, and cardiomyopathy: a newly recognized syndrome.
     Trans.Amer.Ophthal.Soc.1965,63:559–625
6   Kearns,T.P.,Sayre,G.P.
     Retinitis pigmentosa, external ophthalmoplegia and complete
     heart block. Unusual syndrome with histologic study in one
     of two cases.
     Arch.Ophthal.1958,20:280–289
7   McLeod,J.G.,Baker,W.deC.,Shorey,C.D.,Kerr,C.B.
     Mitochondrial myopathy with multisystem abnormalities
     and normal ocular movements.
     J.neurol.Sci.1975,24:39–52
8   Morgan-Hughes,J.A.,Mair,W.G.P.
     Atypical muscle mitochondria in oculoskeletal myopathy.
     Brain 1973,96:215–224
9   Okamura,K.,Santa,T.,Nagae,K.,Omae,T.
     Congenital oculoskeletal myopathy with abnormal muscle
     and liver mitochondria.
     J.neurol.Sci.1976,27:79–91
10   Olson,W.,Engel,W.K.,Walsh,G.O.,Einaugler,R.
     Oculocraniosomatic neuromuscular disease with 'ragged-red'
     fibers. Histochemical and ultrastructural changes in limb
     muscles of a group of patients with idiopathic progressive
     external ophthalmoplegia.
     Arch.Neurol.(Chic.)1972,26:193–211
11   Schneck,L.,Adachi,M.,Briet,P.,Wolintz,A.,Volk,B.W.
     Ophthalmoplegia plus with morphological and chemical
     studies of cerebellar and muscle tissue.
     J.neurol.Sci.1973,19:37–44
12   Shy,G.M.,Silberberg,D.H.,Appel,S.H.,Mishkin,M.M.,
     Godfrey,E.H.
     A generalized disorder of nervous system, skeletal muscle
     and heart resembling Refsum's disease and Hurler's

syndrome. I. Clinical, pathological and biochemical characteristics.
Amer.J.Med.1967,42:163–168

13   Tamura,K.,Santa,T.,Kuroiwa,Y.
Familial oculocranioskeletal neuromuscular disease with abnormal muscle mitochondria.
Brain1974,97:665–672

14   Zintz,R.,Villiger,W.
Elektronenmikroskopische Befunde bei 3 Fällen von chronisch progressiver okulärer Muskeldystrophie.
Ophthalmologica 1967,153:439–459

Congenital myopathies

There is an increasing amount of literature on congenital myopathies named after a peculiar morphological abnormality as seen by light or electron microscopy. Most of these myopathies have a more or less identical clinical picture that can be summarized as follows:

The patients show a marked generalized hypotonia after birth (floppy babies).

Congenital skeletal abnormalities, for instance a high arched palate, a long face, hip dislocation or pes cavus, are frequently present. They have delayed motor milestones and when they start to walk they tend to fall easily and are never able to run or jump. There is no, or only very slow, progression of the disorder. On examination, muscular weakness is usually widespread but more marked proximally, and associated with thinness of the muscle bulk and decreased or absent deep tendon reflexes. In some instances facial weakness or involvement of the extra-ocular muscles is present. The activity of serum creatine phosphokinase is normal or mildly increased. The electromyogram shows short-duration, small-amplitude and polyphasic motor unit potentials. The motor nerve conduction velocities are normal.

Muscle biopsy reveals in many cases a type I fibre predominance (or: type II fibre paucity).

In addition to congenital distal myopathy (page 52) and congenital
dystrophia myotonica (page 153), the following congenital myopathies
were recognized, mainly because of the histopathological findings:
Central core disease (page 71)
Centronuclear myopathy (page 80)
Congenital fibre type disproportion (page 89)
Congenital lipid storage disease (page 217)
Congenital mitochondria-lipid-glycogen disease (page 217)
Congenital muscular dystrophy (page 91)
Focal loss of cross-striations (page 93)
Minicore disease (page 96)
Multicore disease (page 95)
Myopathy with lysis of myofibrils (page 100)
Myotubular myopathy (page 80)
Nemaline myopathy (page 103)
Reducing body myopathy (page 112)
Type I fibre atrophy and myotube-like structures (page 114)
Type I fibre hypotrophy with central nuclei (page 81)

Other congenital myopathies were named after some special features as
seen by electron microscopy:
Congenital myopathies with abnormal mitochondria (page 122)
Fingerprint body myopathy (page 115)
Sarcotubular myopathy (page 117)
Zebra body myopathy (page 119)

The rods (page 110), seen in nemaline myopathy, were found in many other neuromuscular diseases. The presence of rods in a biopsy together with cores, with focal loss of cross-striations or with disproportion of fibre types, has been observed.

Abundant central nuclei were not only seen in centronuclear or myotubular myopathies, but also in myopathies with lysis of myofibrils or with disproportion of fibre types. Focal loss of cross-striations as seen in the congenital myopathy bearing this name, were also found together with the lesions usually observed in multicore disease. All these histopathological changes, together with fingerprint bodies, zebra bodies or mitochondrial abnormalities, appeared to be non-specific reactions of the muscle fibre.

Late onset types of nemaline myopathy, centronuclear and myotubular myopathy, were also described.

Moreover, several different modes of hereditary transmission were recognized.

Therefore, classification is impossible on clinical, morphological or genetic grounds.

Although all the names, based on pathological findings, have given rise to much confusion, no better alternative is at present available for the description of the congenital myopathies.

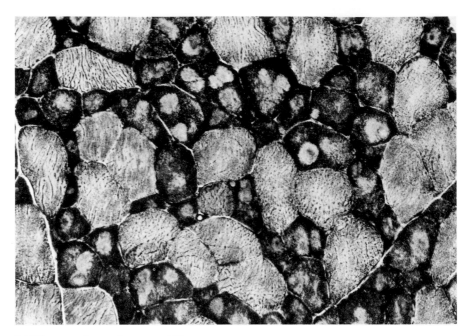

NADH-tetrazolium reductase, ×150

Cores are collections of abnormally stained myofibrils running along the whole length of the muscle fibre. In transverse sections one, or sometimes several (up to five) cores can be seen. The core region shows no activity of oxidative enzymes and phosphorylase and is unstained by reactions for glycogen or lipid.

The myofibrillar ATPase activity of the core is normal or decreased.

The figure shows a transverse section of a muscle biopsy from a patient suffering from central core disease (page 71), stained for the activity of NADH-tetrazolium reductase. The cores are present only in the (darker stained) type I fibres and are devoid of enzyme activity. Many of the cores have an eccentric position, while some fibres contain two cores.

Electron microscopy of the core region shows closely packed myofibrils and reduction or absence of glycogen particles, mitochondria and sarcoplasmic reticulum. The sarcomeres of the core area are slightly contracted compared to those of the non-core region. Within the core, small foci displaying streaming or a zig-zag pattern of the Z discs are found.

Not every core in central core disease has a central position and not every patient with cores in the muscle biopsy is suffering from central core disease.

In 1956, Shy and Magee [27] described a family of 5 patients through three generations, with a probable autosomal dominantly inherited, non-progressive myopathy.

The disease was either congenital or developed within the first months of life.

Hypotonia was evident in the children and the motor development was retarded.

Wasting was not a prominent feature. Examination revealed primary proximal weakness, more severe in the lower extremities. Weakness of the orbicularis muscles was observed in one patient. Four of the patients had pes planus. The deep tendon reflexes were normally active. The only abnormal laboratory finding was excessive urinary creatine excretion and decreased creatinine excretion.

Muscle biopsies showed a collection of abnormal myofibrils in the centre of nearly every muscle fibre; these fibrils stained azurophilically with the Gomori trichrome stain, whereas the outer fibrils stained a normal red. Some fibres contained several — as many as five — bundles of abnormal myofibrils. Longitudinal sections revealed such fibrils running almost the entire length of the fibre. There was an increase of internal nuclei and fat tissue. In one case only a few fibres were abnormal.

The name central core disease was given to this myopathy [15].

Since then, many reports have been published, in which the disease was either sporadic [3–4,5,12,18,20,22,25], inherited as an autosomal dominant [1,9,17,26] or probably autosomal recessive [8] trait.

The clinical picture is that of hypotonia and marked delay in motor milestones in infancy. There is weakness affecting the muscles of the pelvic girdle and legs more than the shoulder girdle and arms, and affecting the proximal muscles more than the distal. Occasionally, there may be facial weakness [3,4,12,20,21,27]. The severity of the mainly non-progressive weakness is variable: usually it is mild. Some patients had no complaints [9,26] or even no muscular weakness [28].

Congenital hip dislocation [1,2,4,14,26] and other skeletal deformities, such as kyphoscoliosis, lumbar lordosis, pes planus and pes cavus, are relatively frequent [17,28].

The deep tendon reflexes may be normal, decreased or absent.

The activity of serum creatine phosphokinase is normal or slightly increased [22,26].

The electromyogram shows short-duration, small-amplitude and polyphasic motor unit potentials in most cases, but polyphasic potentials of normal [22] or long [17] duration and increased voltage have been described. Motor nerve conduction velocities are normal.

In transverse sections of the muscle fibres one, or sometimes several, cores are seen in the centre or in the periphery of the fibres (page 70). The core region is devoid of oxidative enzyme and phosphorylase activities and glycogen. The cores may display a normal or diminished myofibrillar ATPase activity. In longitudinal sections it is seen that the core can be followed along the whole length of the fibre.

In many biopsies there is a type I fibre predominance [2,4,9,17,21,24] but a normal mosaic of type I and type II fibres may be seen [4,6,9].

Both forms of distribution of fibre types may be found in affected members of the same family [9]. In the majority of the biopsies the cores were present in the type I fibres only, although cores were also present in type II C fibres [7,23].

There is one report on a sporadic case with cores restricted to the type II fibres [25].

The percentage of fibres with cores can vary from a few per cent to almost 100 per cent. This may vary within affected members of the same family [9,14,16].

In one family, the biopsy of the mother showed type I fibre predominance and cores in 45 per cent of the type I fibres. The biopsies of her two affected children showed type I predominance without any cores [21].

There is no relationship between the clinical manifestations or severity of the muscular weakness and the number of fibres containing cores.

Electron microscopy of the core region reveals closely packed myofibrils and a marked reduction or absence of mitochondria, glycogen particles and sarcotubules. There are small foci where the Z bands are widened and show streaming or a zig-zag pattern. When there is marked distortion of the cross-banding pattern, while the individual myofibrils are poorly defined, this has been called unstructured core [23].

Rods (page 110) have been found in the muscle fibres of patients suffering from central core disease [17,23], and also in a patient with pes cavus, without muscle weakness, type I fibre predominance and cores in the type I fibres [28].
Rods and central cores were present in a muscle biopsy from a patient suffering from a congenital non-progressive myopathy. The muscle biopsy of her affected daughter showed only cores [1]. Cores were also seen in the muscle fibres of a patient suffering from nemaline myopathy [19].
These observations suggest a close relationship in the formation of these two non-specific, structural alterations of the muscle fibre.

Muscle phosphorylase activity was found to be reduced in a patient and his non-affected father [12]. In the patient, this might have been related to the predominance of type I fibres that are normally poor in phosphorylase activity, but it remained unexplained in the father. On the other hand, a patient with central core disease and type I fibre predominance showed normal muscle phosphorylase activity, while her affected father, with the same histological and histochemical features, had a reduced activity [17].

It has been proposed that central core disease represents an abnormality of the neural influence during embryonic differentiation of the muscle fibres [10,13]. This neurogenic hypothesis is based on morphological similarities of the cores to target and targetoid fibres, on the type I fibre predominance and on the formation of core-like fibres in cat soleus muscle fibres 3–5 weeks following total denervation [11]. This hypothesis is also supported by the finding of an increase in the terminal innervation ratio as reported in several patients [16,17,28].

Patients suffering from central core disease may develop malignant hyperpyrexia [6,16]. Consequently, great care must be taken in a patient suffering from this disease when operations are taken into consideration, for instance for pes cavus.

References 1   Afifi,A.K.,Smith,J.W.,Zellweger,H.
Congenital nonprogressive myopathy. Central core disease and nemaline myopathy in one family.
Neurology(Minneap.)1965,15:371–381

2   Armstrong,R.M.,Koenigsberger,R.,Mellinger,J.,Lovelace,R.E.
Central core disease with congenital hip dislocation: study of two families.
Neurology(Minneap.)1971,21:369–376

3   Bethlem,J.,PosthumusMeyjes,F.E.
Congenital, non-progressive central core disease of Shy and Magee.
Psychiat.Neurol.Neurochir.1960,63:246–251

4   Bethlem,J.,VanWijngaarden,G.K.,Meijer,A.E.F.H.,Fleury,P.
Observations on central core disease.
J.neurol.Sci.1971,14:293–299

5   Brooke,M.H.,Neville,H.E.,Armstrong,J.
Central core disease: ten new cases with a histochemical variation in one.
Neurology(Minneap.)1970,20:386

6   Denborough,M.A.,Dennett,X.,Anderson,R.M.
Central-core disease and malignant hyperpyrexia.
Brit.med.J.1973,1:272–273

7   Dubowitz,V.,Brooke,M.H.
Muscle Biopsy: a modern approach.
London,Saunders,1973

8   Dubowitz,V.,Platts,M.
Central core disease of muscle with focal wasting.
J.Neurol.Neurosurg.Psychiat.1965,28:432–437

9   Dubowitz,V.,Roy,S.
Central core disease of muscle: clinical, histochemical and electron microscopic studies of an affected mother and child.
Brain 1970,93:133-146

10   Engel,W.K.
A critique of congenital myopathies and other disorders.
In:Exploratory Concepts in Muscular Dystrophy and
Related Disorders.Proceedings of the International Conference
Convened by Muscular Dystrophy Associations of America,
Harriman,New York,October22–27,1966.A.T.Milhorat(ed.).
Amsterdam,Excerpta Medica,1967,pp.27–40.(Int.Congr.
Ser.147)

11   Engel,W.K.,Brooke,M.H.,Nelson,P.G.
Histochemical studies of denervated or tenotomized cat
muscle: illustrating difficulties in relating experimental
animal conditions to human neuromuscular diseases.
Ann.N.Y.Acad.Sci.1966,138:160–185

12   Engel,W.K.,Foster,J.B.,Hughes,B.P.,Huxley,H.E.,Mahler,R.
Central core disease – an investigation of a rare muscle
cell abnormality.
Brain 1961,84:167–185

13   Engel,W.K.,Warmolts,J.R.
The motor unit. Diseases affecting it in toto or in portio.
In:New Developments in Electromyography and Clinical
Neurophysiology,Vol.1.J.E.Desmedt(ed.).Basel,Karger,1973.
pp.141–177

14   Gonatas,N.K.,Perez,M.C.,Shy,G.M.,Evangelista,I.
Central 'core' disease of skeletal muscle. Ultrastructural
and cytochemical observations in two cases.
Amer.J.Path.1965,47:503–524

15   Greenfield,J.G.,Cornman,T.,Shy,G.M.
The prognostic value of the muscle biopsy in the 'floppy infant'.
Brain 1958,81:461–484

16   Isaacs,H.,Barlow,M.B.
Central core disease associated with elevated creatine
phosphokinase levels. Two members of a family known
to be susceptible to malignant hyperpyrexia.
S.A.med.J.1974,48:640–642

17   Isaacs,H.,Heffron,J.J.A.,Badenhorst,M.
Central core disease. A correlated genetic, histochemical,
ultramicroscopic, and biochemical study.
J.Neurol.Neurosurg.Psychiat.1975,38:1177–1186

18   Jean,R.,Bonnet,H.,Pages,A.,Cadilhac,J.,Baldet,P.,Dumas,R.
Myopathie congénitale non progressive avec axe central
(central core disease).
Arch.franç.Pédiat.1971,28:65–82

19   Karpati,G.,Carpenter,S.,Andermann,F.
A new concept of childhood nemaline myopathy.
Arch.Neurol.(Chic.)1971,24:291–304

20   Mittelbach,F.,Pongratz,D.
Klinische,histologische und histochemische Untersuchungen
über einen Fall von Central Core Disease
(Zentralfibrillenmyopathie).
Dtsch.Z.Nervenheilk.1968,194:232–242

21   Morgan-Hughes,J.A.,Brett,E.M.,Lake,B.D.,Tomé,F.M.S.
Central core disease or not? Observations on a family
with a non-progressive myopathy.
Brain 1973,96:527–536

22   Mrozek,K.,Strugalska,M.,Fidzianska,A.
A sporadic case of central core disease.
J.neurol.Sci.1970,10:339–348

23   Neville,H.E.,Brooke,M.H.
Central core fibers: structured and unstructured.
In:Basic Research in Myology.Proceedings of the
2nd International Congress on Muscle Diseases,
Perth,22–26 November 1971.Part1.B.A.Kakulas(ed.).
Amsterdam,Excerpta Medica,1973,pp.497–511.
(Int.Congr.Ser.294)

24   Pascual-Castroviejo,I.,Gutiérrez,M.,Rodríguez-Costa,T.,
López-Martín,V.,Ricoy,J.M.,Morales,M.C.
'Central core disease'. Presentación de cuatro casos y revisión
de la literatura.
An.esp.Pediat.1974,7:524–536

25   Pongratz,D.,Heuser,M.,Koppenwallner,C.,Hübner,G.
Central core disease mit 'structured cores' in Typ II-Fasern.
Klin.Wschr.1976,54:117–122

26   Ramsey,P.L.,Hensinger,R.N.
Congenital dislocation of the hip associated with central core
disease.
J.Bone Jt.Surg.1975,57-A:648–651

27 Shy,G.M.,Magee,K.R.
A new congenital non-progressive myopathy.
Brain 1956,79:610–621

28 Telerman-Toppet,N.,Gérard,J.M.,Coërs,C.
Central core disease. A study of clinically unaffected muscle.
J.neurol.Sci.1973,19:207–223

In 1966, Bethlem, Van Gool, Hülsmann and Meijer [2] described a family
of 3 patients, through three generations, suffering from a non-progressive
myopathy and muscle cramps following exercise, with cores in the muscle
fibres. The disease was inherited as an autosomal dominant trait.

There was no hypotonia after birth and no delay of the motor development.
Running and climbing stairs, however, had always been difficult because
they resulted in stiffening of the leg muscles. The patients described this
stiffness as a painless, or almost painless, cramp of the muscles. The stiffness disappeared after a few minutes rest. The cramps could easily be elicited
by vigorous exertion, which produced within one minute stiffness and
hardening of the muscles concerned.

On examination, there was only mild proximal weakness without wasting,
particularly of the lower limbs. Other affected members of this family
showed kyphoscoliosis and congenital hip dislocation [1]. The deep tendon reflexes were normally active and symmetrical.

Electromyography showed short-duration, low-amplitude motor unit
potentials.

Muscle biopsies revealed cores in the type I fibres (page 70) in all three
patients, while rods were seen by light microscopy in two cases and by
electron microscopy in the other case [1]. In one of the biopsies, the centre
of the cores frequently contained a zone with greatly increased enzyme
activity and with relatively increased glycogen. In another biopsy, the
terminal innervation ratio was normal [3].

The clinical picture of the disorder being entirely different from that of
central core disease, the condition was considered to be a new disease
with cores.

References 1 Bethlem,J.
Unpublished observations.
2 Bethlem,J.,VanGool,J.,Hülsmann,W.C.,Meyer,A.E.F.H.
Familial non-progressive myopathy with muscle cramps
after exercise. A new disease associated with cores in
the muscle fibres.

Brain 1966,89:569–588

3 Coërs,C.,Telerman-Toppet,N.,Gérard,J.M.,Szliwowski,H.,
Bethlem,J.,VanWijngaarden,G.K.
Changes in motor innervation and histochemical pattern
of muscle fibers in some congenital myopathies.
Neurology(Minneap.)1976,26:1046–1053

The first description of a case belonging to this group of diseases was given in 1966 by Spiro, Shy and Gonatas [29]. The patient was a 12-year-old boy with normal labour and perinatal events. At 3 months of age he was unable to lift his head while in the prone position. In the next three months there was progressive vomiting and irritability followed by an operation for bilateral subdural haemotoma. At that time bilateral ptosis was noted. The child walked at 17 months but was never able to run. He developed a slowly progressive generalized muscular weakness, probably starting in the lower limbs.

Examination revealed bilateral ptosis and limitation of the movements of the extra-ocular muscles, facial diplegia and generalized weakness, more pronounced in the distal than the proximal muscles, with absent deep tendon reflexes. The serum creatine phosphokinase activity was mildly increased.

Electromyographic investigations were equivocal.

Two biopsies of the gastrocnemius muscle were taken within an interval of approximately 3 years. In the first biopsy about 85 per cent of the muscle fibres contained 1–4 internal nuclei; in the majority of these fibres there was an absence of subsarcolemmic nuclei. Surrounding the centrally placed nuclei there were areas devoid of myofibrils.

In the second biopsy, about 45 per cent of the muscle fibres showed these changes.

Histochemical studies revealed an absence of myofibrillar ATPase activity and an increased or decreased oxidative enzyme activity in the perinuclear zones.

Electron microscopy showed, in the areas adjacent to the central nuclei, no myofibrils but aggregates of mitochondria.

These abnormal fibres were thought to have the characteristic appearance of myotubes ordinarily found in early fetal life. It was postulated that the finding of myotubes in the muscle tissue of an adolescent boy indicated an arrest in development of the muscle at a cellular level.

Because of the presence of myotubes in the biopsies, the disease was called myotubular myopathy.

One year later Sher, Rimalovski, Athanassiades and Aronson [27] described two sisters suffering from a slowly progressive myopathy with onset in the first years of life. The immediate post-natal period had been un-remarkable.

On examination, generalized muscular weakness and wasting, including ptosis and limitation of the eye movements, was found.

Muscle biopsies revealed central nuclei in 50–84 per cent of the fibres in cross-sections and 80–98 per cent of the fibres in longitudinal sections.

The mother showed mild bilateral ptosis and had central nuclei in 29 per cent of the fibres in cross-sections and 39 per cent in longitudinal sections. It was proposed that the disorder was transmitted as an autosomal reces-sive trait.

Because of the uncertainty about the pathogenesis of the disease, the more descriptive name familial centronuclear myopathy was suggested.

These reports were followed by many other publications, in which the au-thors either used the name myotubular myopathy [2,8,16] or centronuclear myopathy [3,5,11–13,19,20,24,25] or both [21–23,30]. Some authors called the disease myotubular myopathy in one publication, but preferred the name centronuclear myopathy in a subsequent publication on the same patients [8,21,27,28]. The name peri-centronuclear myopathy [7] has been used once, but it has never been adopted by other authors.

In addition it was found that in some biopsies there was also smallness of type I fibres [2,8,12,20] and this led to still other designations such as type I fibre atrophy and central nuclei [15] or, probably more rightly, type I fibre hypotrophy with central nuclei [6,9,10,14]. In one case, sub-typing of type I fibres showed that all hypotrophic fibres with central nuclei belonged to the sub-type 1 B [1].

Finally, there were reports on congenital myopathies with type I fibre atrophy or hypotrophy without any other pathological features [17,26].

The relationship of these histopathological findings was suggested by the observation on a non-progressive myopathy in a mother and her daugh-ter [18].

The mother showed selective atrophy of type I fibres, the daughter had central nuclei, surrounded by areas devoid of any enzyme activities, in approximately 50 per cent of both fibre types.

In another observation on a slowly progressive myopathy with onset in early childhood, muscle biopsy revealed type I fibre atrophy, central nuclei in both fibre types, as well as occasional fibres with a large central area devoid of myofibrils and containing central nuclei [4].

It soon became apparent that the patients with these kind of histopathological changes in their biopsies were suffering from a variety of conditions with different clinical and genetic features:

Many cases were congenital and presented as floppy infants, but onset was sometimes later in childhood [4,5,13,16,25,27] or in adult life [11,20,30]. Ptosis and weakness of extra-ocular and facial muscles, though present in the first reports, appeared to be absent in about half the patients.

Sporadic occurrence, as well as transmission as an autosomal recessive, autosomal dominant or X-linked recessive trait, have all been reported.

References   1   Askanas,V.,Engel,W.K.
Distinct subtypes of type I fibers of human skeletal muscle.
Neurology(Minneap.)1975,25:879–887

2   Badurska,B.,Fidzianska,A.,Kamieniecka,Z.,Prot,J.,
Strugalska,H.
Myotubular myopathy.
J.neurol.Sci.1969,8:563–571

3   Bethlem,J.,Meyer,A.E.F.H.,Schellens,J.P.M.,Vroom,J.J.
Centronuclear myopathy.
Europ.Neurol.1968,1:325–333

4   Bethlem,J.,VanWijngaarden,G.K.,Mumenthaler,M.,
Meyer,A.E.F.H.
Centronuclear myopathy with type I fiber atrophy and
'myotubes'.
Arch.Neurol.(Chic.)1970,23:70–73

5   Bradley,W.G.,Price,D.L.,Watanabe,C.K.
Familial centronuclear myopathy.
J.Neurol.Neurosurg.Psychiat.1970,33:687–693

6   Brooke,M.H.,Williamson,T.
         An adult case of type I muscle fiber hypotrophy: an
         abnormality of monosynaptic reflex function.
         Neurology(Minneap.)1969,19:280

7   Campbell,M.J.,Rebeiz,J.J.,Walton,J.N.
         Myotubular, centronuclear or peri-centronuclear myopathy?
         J.neurol.Sci.1969,8:425–443

8   Coleman,R.F.,Thompson,L.R.,Niehuis,A.W.,Munsat,T.L.,
         Pearson,C.M.
         Histochemical investigation of 'myotubular' myopathy.
         Arch.Path.1968,86:365–376

9   Engel,W.K.
         Selective and nonselective susceptibility of muscle fiber types.
         A new approach to human neuromuscular diseases.
         Arch.Neurol.(Chic.)1970,22:97–117

10   Engel,W.K.,Gold,G.N.,Karpati,G.
         Type I fiber hypotrophy and central nuclei. A rare
         congenital muscle abnormality with a possible experimental
         model.
         Arch.Neurol.(Chic.)1968,18:435–444

11   Goulon,M.,Fardeau,M.,Got,C.,Babinet,P.,Manko,E.
         Myopathie centro-nucléaire d'expression clinique tardive.
         Etude clinique, histologique et ultrastructurale d'une nouvelle
         observation.
         Rev.Neurol.1976,132:275–290

12   Harriman,D.G.F., Haleem,M.A.
         Centronuclear myopathy in old age.
         J.Pathol.1972,108:237–248

13   Headington,J.T.,McNamara,J.O.,Brownell,A.K.
         Centronuclear myopathy: histochemistry and electron
         microscopy. Report of two cases.
         Arch.Path.1975,99:16–24

14   Inokuchi,T.,Umezaki,H.,Santa,T.
         A case of type I muscle fibre hypotrophy and internal nuclei.
         J.Neurol.Neurosurg.Psychiat.1975,38:475–482

15   Karpati,G.,Carpenter,S.,Nelson,R.F.
         Type I muscle fibre atrophy and central nuclei. A rare familial
         neuromuscular disease.
         J.neurol.Sci.1970,10:489–500

16 Kinoshita,M.,Cadman,T.E.
Myotubular myopathy.
Arch.Neurol.(Chic.)1968,18:265–271

17 Kinoshita,M.,Satoyoshi,E.,Kumagai,M.
Familial type I fiber atrophy.
J.neurol.Sci.1975,25:11–17

18 Kinoshita,M.,Satoyoshi,E.,Matsuo,N.
'Myotubular myopathy' and 'type I fiber atrophy' in a family.
J.neurol.Sci.1975,26:575–582

19 Lolova,I.,Bojinova,T.,Kilimov,N.,Gerehev,A.
A case of centronuclear myopathy.
Z.Neurol.1973,205:83–90

20 McLeod,J.G.,Baker,W.deC.,Lethlean,A.K.,Shorey,C.D.
Centronuclear myopathy with autosomal dominant
inheritance.
J.neurol.Sci.1972,15:375–387

21 Munsat,T.L.,Thompson,L.R.,Coleman,R.F.
Centronuclear ('myotubular') myopathy.
Arch.Neurol.(Chic.)1969,20:120–131

22 OrtizdeZarate,J.C.,Maruffo,A.
The descending ocular myopathy of early childhood
myotubular or centronuclear myopathy.
Europ.Neurol.1970,3:1–12

23 Pascual-Castroviejo,I.,Ricoy,J.R.
Miopatía miotubular o centronuclear. (Presentación de
dos casos y revisíon de la literatura).
An.esp.Pediat.1974,7:537–550

24 Pongratz,D.,Heuser,M.,Mittelbach,F.,Struppler,A.
Die sogenannte congenitale centronucleäre Myopathie —
eine primäre Neuropathie?
Acta neuropath.1975,32:9–19

25 SchochetJr,S.S.,Zellweger,H.,Ionasescu,V.,McCormick,W.F.
Centronuclear myopathy: disease entity or a syndrome?
Light- and electron-microscopic study of two cases and
review of the literature.
J.neurol.Sci.1972,16:215–228

26 Serratrice,G.,Pellissier,J.F.,Gastaut,J.L.,Pouget,J.
Myopathie congénitale avec hypotrophie sélective des fibres
de type I.

Rev Neurol.1975,131 : 813–815

27   Sher,J.H.,Rimalovski,A.B.,Athanassiades,T.J.,Aronson,S.M.
Familial centronuclear myopathy : a clinical and pathological
study.
Neurology(Minneap.)1967,17:727–742

28   Sher,J.H.,Rimalowski,A.B.,Athanassiades,T.J.,Aronson,S.M.
Familial myotubular myopathy : a clinical, pathological,
histochemical, and ultrastructural study.
J.Neuropath.exp.Neurol.1967,26:132–133

29   Spiro,A.J.,Shy,G.M.,Gonatas,N.K.
Myotubular myopathy. Persistence of fetal muscle in an
adolescent boy.
Arch.Neurol.(Chic.)1966,14:1–14

30   Vital,C.,Vallat,J.-M.,Martin,F.,LeBlanc,M.,Bergouignan,M.
Etude clinique et ultrastructurale d'un cas de myopathie
centronucléaire (myotubular myopathy) de l'adulte.
Rev.Neurol.1970,123:117–130

In 1972, McLeod, Baker, Lethlean and Shorey [2] reported on the first large family in which autosomal dominant inheritance was beyond dispute. In 5 generations 16 members were affected.

Onset was said to be between the ages of 20 and 30 years, but of the 6 patients that could be examined, 4 had noticed muscular weakness in childhood and were never able to run. There was very slow progression and many patients reached an advanced age.

Muscular weakness and wasting were present predominantly in the proximal muscles, but in some cases facial and distal muscles were also involved. Slight ptosis was present in only one patient and no limitation of the eye movements was observed. The deep tendon reflexes were absent or reduced.

Serum creatine phosphokinase activity was normal. The electromyogram showed polyphasic motor units potentials of short duration and with low amplitudes. Motor and sensory nerve conduction velocities were normal.

Muscle biopsies showed type I fibre smallness and central nuclei in about 60 per cent of both type I and type II fibres. Electron microscopy demonstrated no zone of sarcoplasm between the central nuclei and the surrounding fibrils.

The clinical features resembled those of another, probably autosomal dominant disease, in which there was type I fibre smallness and central nuclei mainly in the type I fibres [1].

References 1   Karpati,G.,Carpenter,S.,Nelson,R.F.
Type I muscle fibre atrophy and central nuclei. A rare familial neuromuscular disease.
J.neurol.Sci.1970,10:489–500

2   McLeod,J.G.,Baker,W.deC.,Lethlean,A.K.,Shorey,C.D.
Centronuclear myopathy with autosomal dominant inheritance.
J.neurol.Sci.1972,15:375–387

In 1969, Van Wijngaarden, Fleury, Bethlem and Meijer [5] described an X-linked recessive congenital myopathy, in which there was severe hypotonia and respiratory insufficiency with cyanosis at birth. This sometimes resulted in early death. If the boy survived this phase, more or less generalized muscular weakness persisted, with the extra-ocular, facial and neck muscles always affected. There was little or no progression. The deep tendon reflexes were usually absent. The serum creatine phosphokinase activity was normal, or slightly elevated in the older patients. Electromyographic investigations were equivocal. The motor nerve conduction velocities were normal.

Muscle histopathology was variable, but the most characteristic feature was the presence of small muscle fibres with a peripheral rim of myofibrils and a central zone in which a collection of sarcoplasmic components, and sometimes also a central nucleus, was seen. These fibres had the morphological and histochemical characteristics of myotubes as seen in fetal muscle. However, it could not be proven that the fibres were the result of an arrest in muscle development and therefore represented persistent fetal myotubes. Therefore, they were not called myotubes but 'myotubes' between quotation marks. A few of these fibres were also seen in the muscle biopsies of 2 of 3 known carriers.

The authors stressed the striking histopathological similarity between their cases and the case described by Engel, Gold and Karpati [2] that was named type I fibre hypotrophy and central nuclei. This male patient was born apnoeic and suffered from atelectasis of the right lung for which he required oxygen during three days. Crying and swallowing were weak; there was severe general weakness and hypotonia, but the facial and extra-ocular muscles were not affected.

In 1974, Meyers, Golomb, Hansen and McKusick [4] reported on the brother of this patient who had similar clinical and morphological features. The pedigree suggested an X-linked recessive mode of inheritance.

A second, non-related family was described from The Netherlands [1] in which decreased fetal movements and hydramnios were additional findings. In this family the expression of the disease was more severe and all patients died, usually within 1–2 days after birth, from alveolar hypoventilation due to insufficient lung expansion.

Carriers could be recognized by the presence of scattered 'myotubes' and small type I fibres in their biopsies.

The pathogenesis of the disorder remains obscure. In two cases no abnormalities were found in the spinal cord [1,5], while the terminal innervation ratio was normal in one patient [3].

References   1   Barth,P.G.,VanWijngaarden,G.K.,Bethlem,J.
                       X-linked myotubular myopathy with fatal neonatal asphyxia.
                       Neurology(Minneap.)1975,25:531–536
                  2   Engel,W.K.,Gold,G.N.,Karpati,G.
                       Type I fiber hypotrophy and central nuclei. A rare congenital
                       muscle abnormality with a possible experimental model.
                       Arch.Neurol.(Chic.)1968,18:435–444
                  3   Coërs,C.,Telerman-Toppet,N.,Gérard,J.M.,Szliwowski,H.,
                       Bethlem,J.,VanWijngaarden,G.K.
                       Changes in motor innervation and histochemical pattern of
                       muscle fibers in some congenital myopathies.
                       Neurology(Minneap.)1976,26:1046–1053
                  4   Meyers,K.R.,Golomb,H.M.,Hansen,J.L.,McKusick,V.A.
                       Familial neuromuscular disease with 'myotubes'.
                       Clin.Genet.1974,5:327–337
                  5   VanWijngaarden,G.K.,Fleury,P.,Bethlem,J.,Meyer,A.E.F.H.
                       Familial 'myotubular' myopathy.
                       Neurology(Minneap.)1969,19:901–908

In 1973, Brooke [1] reported on a group of patients suffering from a disease which he named congenital fibre type disproportion. The main features were generalized muscular weakness and hypotonia, present at birth or shortly after. Many of these floppy babies showed muscle contractures and multiple skeletal abnormalities, such as hip dislocations, kyphoscoliosis, varus and valgus deformities of the feet, and a high arched palate.

The hypotonia and weakness tended to progress during the first two years of life, but after that the clinical features seemed to become stationary or even improved. In the first, severe period, recurrent respiratory infections often developed.

Most patients were abnormally small, with a weight below the 3rd percentile for the age, even though the birth weight was often normal. The height was also decreased below the 10th percentile in about half the patients. Intelligence was normal or above average.

The activity of serum creatine phosphokinase was mildly raised in some patients.

Electromyography showed either no abnormalities or short-duration polyphasic potentials. Conduction velocities were normal in all patients.

Muscle biopsies were characterized by relatively small type I fibres and relatively large type II fibres, particularly type II B fibres. In addition to the disproportion in the size of the fibres, there was also a disproportion in the number of fibres: half of the biopsies showed type I fibre predominance. In some cases additional findings were present, such as an increase in the number of fibres with internal nuclei, moth-eaten fibres and formation of rods.

In this condition — probably more a syndrome than a disease — there was frequently a history of other members of the family suffering from a neuromuscular disease.

The first morphological proof of such a familial character was given in a report on a father and 2 daughters [2]. The father showed no muscular weakness, but he had generalized reduction of muscle bulk and the deep tendon reflexes of the arms were absent. His biopsy showed type I fibre smallness. The myofilaments often ran an irregular course and in addition some rods were seen. The daughters were born as floppy infants and showed type I fibres with a mean diameter at the lower limit of normal, and hypertrophy of type II fibres. Electron microscopy revealed no abnormalities of the muscle fibres or motor end-plates.

When there is a marked increase of internal nuclei, the histopathological differentiation between congenital fibre type disproportion and type I fibre hypotrophy with internal nuclei (page 81) is arbitrary. Also, the clinical and histochemical characteristics of familial type I fibre atrophy [3] were almost identical to those of congenital fibre type disproportion.

References   1   Brooke,M.H.
                       Congenital fiber type dysproportion.
                       In:Clinical Studies in Myology.B.A.Kakulas(ed.).
                       Amsterdam,Excerpta Medica,1973,pp.147–159
              2   Fardeau,M.,Harpey,J.P.,Caille,B.
                       Disproportion congénitale des différents types de fibre
                       musculaire, avec petitesse relative des fibres de type I.
                       Documents morphologiques concernant les biopsies
                       musculaires prélevées chez trois membres d'une même
                       famille.
                       Rev.Neurol.1975,131 : 745–766
              3   Kinoshita,M.,Satoyoshi,E.,Kumagai,M.
                       Familial type I fiber atrophy.
                       J.neurol.Sci.1975,25:11–17

The name congenital muscular dystrophy has been given for a condition in which there was already at birth marked hypotonia, frequently multiple contractures, and more or less generalized muscular weakness [1,2,4,6–10]. The muscles of the pelvic and shoulder girdles and the proximal limbs were predominantly affected, but in many patients involvement of the neck and facial muscles [1] were found. These cases have sometimes been referred to as amyotonia congenita or – when there were congenital contractures – as arthrogryposis multiplex congenita. The latter syndrome, however, can be seen in both neurogenic and myopathic conditions.

Muscle biopsies showed non-specific changes, such as variation in fibre size, some necrotic or basophilic fibres, increase in the number of fibres with internal nuclei, and proliferation of connective tissue. In very few cases were histochemical studies carried out, and these did not reveal any additional information [1].

Sporadic and hereditary cases have been described, and there is a wide variety in clinical features, severity and progression of the disorder. It is likely that congenital muscular dystrophy is a syndrome and it can be expected that with increasing knowledge of the congenital myopathies, this diagnosis will be made less often.

From Japan, there have been several reports on congenital muscular dystrophy in addition to micropolygyria, to which the name congenital cerebromuscular dystrophy has also been given [3,5].

References   1   Donner,M.,Rapola,J.,Somer,H.
             Congenital muscular dystrophy: a clinico-pathological and
             follow-up study of 15 patients.
             Neuropädiatrie 1975,6:239–258
         2   Gubbay,S.S.,Walton,J.N.,Pearce,G.W.
             Clinical and pathological study of a case of congenital
             muscular dystrophy.
             J.Neurol.Neurosurg.Psychiat.1966,29:500–508
         3   Kamoshita,S.,Konishi,Y.,Segawa,M.,Fukuyama,Y.
             Congenital muscular dystrophy as a disease of the central
             nervous system.

Arch.Neurol.(Chic.)1976,33:513–516

4 Ketelsen,U.-P.,Freund-Mölbert,E.,Beckmann,R.
Klinische und ultrastrukturelle Befunde bei kongenitaler
Muskeldystrophie.
Mschr.Kinderheilk.1971,119:586–592

5 Murakami,T.,Konishi,Y.,Takamiya,M.,Tsukagoshi,H.
Congenital muscular dystrophy associated with
micropolygyria – report of two cases.
Acta path.jap.1975,25:599–612

6 Otto,H.F.,Lücking,T.
Congenitale Muskeldystrophie. Licht- und
elektronenmikroskopische Befunde.
Virchows Arch.Abt.A.Path.Anat.1971,352:324–339

7 Short,J.K.
Congenital muscular dystrophy. A case report with
autopsy findings.
Neurology(Minneap.)1963,13:526–530

8 Vallat,J.-M.,Vital,C.,LeBlanc,M.
Les myopathies congénitales.
Bordeaux méd.1972,5:2439–2451

9 Vassella,F.,Mumenthaler,M.,Rossi,E.,Moser,H.,Wiesmann,U.
Die kongenitale Muskeldystrophie.
Dtsch.Z.Nervenheilk.1967,190:349–374

10 Zellweger,H.,Afifi,A.,McCormick,W.F.,Mergner,W.
Benign congenital muscular dystrophy: a special form of
congenital hypotonia.
Clin.Pediat.1967,6:655–663

In 1967, Engel [2] described a 14-year-old girl in whom hypotonia and generalized muscular weakness, with no, or only very slow, progression had been present from birth. The weakness was greater in the proximal limb muscles and there was a slight ptosis and impaired extra-ocular movements. Nearly all deep tendon reflexes were absent. The activity of serum creatine phosphokinase was normal.

The muscle biopsy showed focal lesions displaying loss of cross-striations but preservation of longitudinally arranged myofibrillar material. Multiple internal nuclei were present within and closely surrounding these abnormal regions (page 98). On histochemical examination, enzyme activities and glycogen appeared to be reduced or absent in these areas. There was widespread type I fibre smallness and significant type I fibre predominance.

In the foci, electron microscopy disclosed myofibrillar degeneration with loss of myofilamentous aligment, smearing of Z disc-like substance and diminution or loss of mitochondria.

The disease was called focal loss of cross-striations.

A similar, progressive disorder leading to death, was described as congenital myopathy with target fibres [4,5]. Familial occurrence of the disease in a brother and sister has been observed [6].

It remains uncertain whether the histopathologic alterations in a case of 'segmental myopathy' were comparable with the abnormalities seen in focal loss of cross-striations [3].

Similar lesions present in the disease called focal loss of cross-striations were observed in other myopathies [1]. However, the clinical, histological and histochemical features of the few cases observed so far, show a certain resemblance. Therefore, it remains a probability that focal loss of cross-striations forms a disease entity.

References 1 Bethlem,J.
Unpublished observations.
2 Engel,W.K.
Muscle biopsies in neuromuscular diseases.
Pediat.Clin.N.Amer.1967,14: 963–995
3 Satoyoshi,E.,Kinoshita,M.
An autopsy case of segmental myopathy.
In:Clinical Studies in Myology.B.A.Kakulas(ed.).
Amsterdam,Excerpta Medica,1973,pp.489–495
4 Schotland,D.L.
Congenital myopathy with target fibers.
Trans.Amer.Neurol.Ass.1967,92:107–111
5 Schotland,D.L.
An electron microscopic study of target fibers, targetlike fibers
and related abnormalities in human muscle.
J.Neuropath.exp.Neurol.1969,28:214–228
6 VanWijngaarden,G.K.,Bethlem,J.,Dingemans,K.P.,Coërs,C.,
Telerman-Toppet,N.,Gérard,J.M.
Familial focal loss of cross-striations.
In press.

In 1971, Engel, Gomez and Groover [3] described two patients suffering from a congenital, non-progressive myopathy characterized by a decrease in the mitochondrial population of multiple foci in muscle fibres.

The first patient, a 13-year-old boy, had generalized hypotonia, weakness of the trunk muscles, and moderate proximal and mild distal weakness of the extremity muscles. He revealed a dolicomorphic habitus.

The second patient, an 11-year-old girl, showed mild ptosis and had diffuse weakness, greater in the proximal than in the distal limb muscles, while the upper extremities were weaker than the lower. The patient had atrial and ventricular septal defects, for which she was operated upon. In addition she had thoracic scoliosis, tight heel cords and slight elbow contractures.

In both patients, the deep tendon reflexes were hypoactive. The serum creatine phosphokinase (CPK) and glutamic-oxaloacetic transaminase activities were normal.

Electromyography disclosed short-duration motor unit potentials and normal motor nerve conduction velocities.

Muscle biopsies revealed type I fibre predominance and numerous small, randomly distributed areas in both type I and II muscle fibres in which focal decrease of oxidative enzyme activity and focal myofibrillar degeneration were seen. Not all areas of decreased oxidative enzyme activities displayed loss of cross-striations. The smallest lesions were 5μ in diameter and occurred in any fibre region. Larger lesions, up to 200μ long in one case, varied considerably in shape and size.

Histometric comparison of myofibrillar and mitochondrial lesions revealed that the mitochondrial lesion was present in a higher proportion of the fibres, occurred with greater frequency per unit area in affected fibres, and had a larger mean area than the myofibrillar lesion.

Electron microscopy of the lesions showed decrease of mitochondria. This was followed by streaming of the Z discs, disruption of the A and I filaments of the sarcomeres and decrease of glycogen granules and sarcotubular profiles.

Intramuscular nerves and motor end-plates were normal.

The second report concerned identical twins, born as floppy infants, with generalized muscular weakness and torticollis [4].
The motor milestones were delayed, although by the age of 6 years marked improvement in muscle strength had occurred. Dolichocephaly was present in both patients. The deep tendon reflexes were hypoactive. The serum CPK activity was normal.
Muscle pathology was similar to that of the previous cases, including the observation of the frequent perpendicular orientation of the long axis of the lesions to the long axis of the muscle fibre.

Multicores were also described in a 46-year-old woman who had a 12-year history of gradual onset of progressive proximal weakness [1]. The deep tendon reflexes were absent. The serum CPK activity was slightly elevated.
The electromyogram showed short-duration and small-amplitude motor unit potentials. Nerve conduction velocities were normal.
This disorder was regarded as multicore disease with onset in middle age. However, the presence of multicores is a non-specific finding and at present it would seem more appropriate to assume the existence of several neuromuscular diseases with multicores.

Minicore disease

In 1974, Currie, Noronha and Harriman [2] reported on two patients suffering from a congenital myopathy with a slowly progressive course. Each had a myopathic facies and generalized weakness and wasting, particularly affecting the sternomastoids and proximal limb muscles. Serum creatine phosphokinase activity was normal.
Muscle pathology showed type I fibre predominance and large numbers of minute foci – up to three sarcomeres in length – of mitochondrial loss.

Electron microscopy revealed focal Z band thinning and sarcomere disintegration. The end-plates were enlarged with numerous expansions. Because of the uniformly small size of the lesions, the designation minicore disease was proposed.

To a limited extent similar small focal lesions can be seen in many neuromuscular diseases and in normal subjects [5]. In multicore disease many of the lesions are larger than in minicore disease. From the pathological point of view, the difference between these abnormal zones and those seen in focal loss of cross-striations, is the presence of vesicular nuclei in and around the lesions of the latter (page 98). However, many lesions in focal loss of cross-striations lack these nuclei. Therefore, the morphological differences of multicore disease, minicore disease and focal loss of cross-striations may not be essential.

References   1   Bonnette,H.,Roelofs,R.,Olson,W.H.
                    Multicore disease report of a case with onset in middle age.
                    Neurology(Minneap.)1974,24:1039–1044
             2   Currie,S.,Noronha,M.,Harriman,D.
                    'Minicore' disease.
                    In:IIIrd International Congress on Muscle Diseases.Amsterdam
                    Excerpta Medica,1974,p.12.(Int.Congr.Ser.334)
             3   Engel,A.G.,Gomez,M.R.,Groover,R.V.
                    Multicore disease. A recently recognized congenital myopathy
                    associated with multifocal degeneration of muscle fibers.
                    Proc.Mayo Clin.1971,46:666–681
             4   Heffner,R.,Cohen,M.,Duffner,P.,Daigler,G.
                    Multicore disease in twins.
                    J.Neurol.Neurosurg.Psychiat.1976,39:602–606
             5   Meltzer,H.Y.,Kunci,R.W.,Click,J.,Yang,V.
                    Incidence of Z band streaming and myofibrillar disruptions
                    in skeletal muscle from healthy young people.
                    Neurology(Minneap.)1976,26:853–857

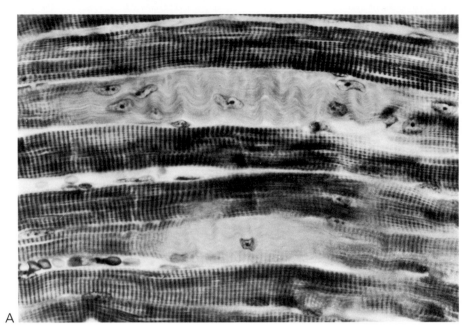

A

PTAH, ×190

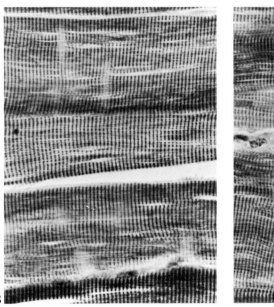

B

PTAH, ×300

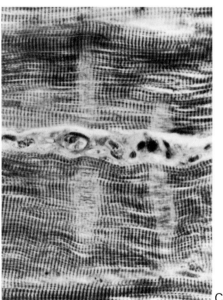

C

PTAH, ×300

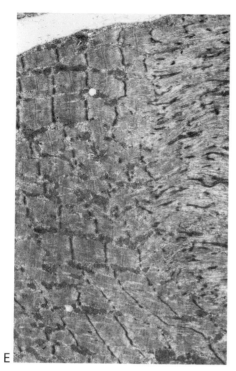
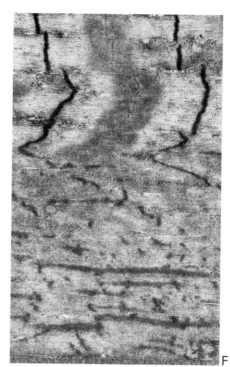

E

F

×1170

×5400; figures kindly supplied by Dr. K.P. Dingemans

In the disorder called focal loss of cross-striations (page 93), the lesions are best seen in sections stained with phosphatungstic acid haematoxylin (PTAH). In and around the abnormal areas, vesicular nuclei with prominent nucleoli are often present (A).

The lesions seen in multicore disease (page 95) do not show these nuclei (B and C). In B the lesions are orientated perpendicular to the long axis of the muscle fibre. Their width is about 5μ. In C, somewhat larger lesions are present, with a width up to 12μ. In these lesions the loss of cross-striations can be clearly seen.

Lesions with and without vesicular nuclei may be present in one biopsy and can be considered as rare but non-specific changes in the muscle fibre. Within the abnormal regions there is no activity of oxidative enzymes, and no glycogen granules or lipid can be seen. Myofibrillar ATPase activity is decreased, while in some lesions the acid phosphatase activity is increased.

Electron microscopy reveals disintegration of the sarcomeres, with streaming of the Z discs and diminution or loss of mitochondria (D). In the demarcation zone there is a zig-zag appearance of the Z discs (E).

Both by light and electron microscopy the very abrupt transition between the normal and abnormal part of the muscle fibre can be observed.

In 1971, Cancilla, Kalyanaraman, Verity, Munsat and Pearson [1] described a 5-year-old girl and her 2-year-old brother, suffering from a non-progressive, or slowly progressive, congenital myopathy with probable lysis of myofibrils in the type I fibres.

The children were born as floppy infants and had delayed motor milestones. On examination, there was hypotonia and generalized muscular weakness, more marked proximally, without wasting. The deep tendon reflexes were normal. The activity of serum creatine phosphokinase was mildly raised. The electromyogram in the girl was reported as normal.

Muscle biopsies revealed type I fibre smallness and type I fibre predominance. The type I fibres showed irregular, usually peripherally located and homogeneous zones without myofibrils or cross-striations. With the myosin ATPase reaction, however, these abnormal zones stained dark. In these areas, sarcolemmal nuclei with prominent nucleoli were present, as well as small vacuoles at the junctional zone between the normal and abnormal parts of the muscle fibre.

Electron microscopy of the abnormal portions showed a uniform, finely granular matrix, with nuclei, scattered mitochondria and glycogen granules. In addition, regions with streaming and disintegration of the Z discs and absence of mitochondria were present. The transitional zone between the normal and abnormal part of the muscle fibre was very abrupt.

The pathological features were considered as a breakdown (lysis) of previously intact myofibrils or as an accumulation of some structural product.

In 1974, Radu, Ionescu, Radu, Paler, Roşu and Marian [5] reported on two cousins, a 5-year-old girl and a 5-year-old boy, with generalized hypotonia and weakness, without wasting, from the first years of life. The girl also had involvement of the extra-ocular muscles.

The deep tendon reflexes were decreased. Activity of the serum creatine phosphokinase was normal. Electromyography suggested a disfunction of the tonic motor units. Muscle biopsies revealed type I fibre smallness (hypotrophy) and an increase of internal nuclei. The type II fibres were of normal size.

The type II fibres, and to a lesser extent the type I fibres, showed homo-
genous central areas in which the myosin ATPase activity was decreased.
The ultrastructural picture of these zones and that of the cases described
above, were considered to be identical.
The mothers were clinically normal, but their muscle biopsies showed
similar histopathological alterations. An autosomal recessive inheritance
of the disorder was assumed.

In 1976, a 5-year-old boy with congenital, non-progressive and generalized
hypotonia and muscular weakness, including the facial muscles, was described by Scelsi, Lanzi, Nespoli and Poggi [6].
Muscle biopsy showed predominance of normal sized type I fibres. There
was a marked reduction in size of the type II fibres. Internal nuclei were
seen in 32 per cent of the type I fibres and 28 per cent of the type II
fibres.
Ultrastructural studies revealed areas with myofibrillar disorientation, frag-
mentation and homogenation of the myofibrils and disintegration of Z disc
material. These were said to be similar to those described in the above
cases.

Preferential type II fibre atrophy is a non-specific phenomenon, which can
develop in cachexia, disuse, chronic corticosteroid intoxication and myasthenia gravis [2]. The above-mentioned ultrastructural changes have
been observed in atrophic type II fibres not only in a patient with type II
muscle fibre hypoplasia [3], but also in patients without neuromuscular
diseases [4].

References   **1**   Cancilla,P.A.,Kalyanaraman,K.,Verity,M.A.,Munsat,T.,
Pearson,C.M.
Familial myopathy with probable lysis of myofibrils in type I
fibers.
Neurology(Minneap.)1971,21:579–585

2   Engel,W.K.
     Selective and non-selective susceptibility of muscle fiber types.
     A new approach to human neuromuscular diseases.
     Arch.Neurol.(Chic.)1970,22:97–117
3   Matsuoka,Y.,Gubbay,S.S.,Kakulas,B.A.
     A new myopathy with type II muscle fibre hypoplasia.
     Proc.Aust.Ass.Neurol.1974,11:155–159
4   Mendell,J.R.,Engel,W.K.
     The fine structure of type II muscle fiber atrophy.
     Neurology(Minneap.)1971,21:358–365
5   Radu,H.,Ionescu,V.,Radu,A.,Paler,V.,Roşu,A.M.,Marian,A.
     Hypotrophic type I muscle fibres with central nuclei, and
     central myofibrillar lysis preferentially involving type II fibres.
     Europ.Neurol.1974,11:108–127
6   Scelsi,R.,Lanzi,G.,Nespoli,L.,Poggi,P.
     Congenital non-progressive myopathy with type II fibre atrophy
     and internal nuclei.
     Europ.Neurol.1976,14:285–293

Nemaline myopathy is also called rod myopathy or rod disease. It was first described in 1963 in two independent publications on a new congenital myopathy.

The first report was that of Shy, Engel, Somers and Wanko [29] who described a 4-year-old girl born as a floppy baby, with subsequent delayed motor development.

Examination revealed generalized hypotonia and muscular weakness, especially of the shoulder and pelvic girdles. The muscles were of lesser bulk than normal, while the tendon reflexes were absent.

Muscle biopsy showed rod-like or thread-like structures in 46 per cent of all muscle fibres. The rods usually occupied the entire length of the involved fibres and could be found either in the subsarcolemmal regions or in the centre of the fibre. The disorder was named nemaline myopathy, after the Greek word for thread (nèma).

In the second report, Conen, Murphy and Donohue [4] described a 4-year-old boy with a similar history and the same clinical features as that of the above-mentioned patient, In addition he showed weakness of the facial, tongue and pharynx muscles, a high palate and a prominent pigeon chest. Muscle biopsy revealed in many fibres rod-shaped formations, termed 'myogranules'. This name has never been adopted by other authors.

The mothers of patients suffering from nemaline myopathy often maintain that the fetal movements were decreased. At birth, the child has the typical clinical picture of a floppy infant. Due to the muscular weakness, resperatory disfunction with cyanosis and difficulties with suckling and swallowing are frequently present in the post-natal period. Aspiration and respiratory infections are the most frequent cause of death [3,20,28].

On inspection the baby shows a myopathic facies, with normal eye movements.

There is skeletal dismorphism, such as an elongated face, high-arched palate, prognathism, malocclusion of the teeth and pigeon chest [17,26]. These findings are rather characteristic but not specific for nemaline myopathy and may also be seen in other congenital myopathies. The muscles are slender and under-developed, giving the impression of generalized muscle hypoplasia. The motor milestones are delayed.

On examination, generalized muscular weakness may be found, mainly involving the proximal and axial muscles, while the extensors of the feet may also be affected [19,25]. The deep tendon reflexes are usually decreased or absent. Kyphoscoliosis and pes cavus may be found. There is no, or only slight, progression [11,16] of the muscular weakness.

It should be stressed that not all patients present this rather severe clinical picture. Symptomatology may be unremarkable and some patients are hardly aware of their muscular deficiency [14].

Serum creatine phosphokinase activity is within normal limits, only very rarely is it mildly raised [2]. Electromyography shows, in most cases, brief-duration, small-amplitude, abundant and polyphasic motor unit potentials. In about 75 per cent of the published cases muscle biopsy showed type I fibre predominance. In the other biopsies a normal mosaic of type I and type II fibres was present. In about half the cases type I fibre smallness was found.

Collections of rods are seen in the subsarcolemmal and central regions of the muscle fibres. They are most easily detected in cryostate sections stained with the modified trichrome stain of Engel and Cunningham [8]. With this method, the rods are stained bright red. Usually vesicular nuclei with prominent nucleoli are present in and around the aggregates of rods.

The number of fibres containing rods differs from case to case, from muscle to muscle in the same patient, and from one part to the other part in the same muscle [16,21,28]. In some biopsies almost 100 per cent of the fibres may contain rods, while other biopsies may even show no rods at all [25]. There is no relationship between the severity of the disease or the muscular weakness on the one hand and the number of fibres with rods on the other.

Although most authors did not find rods in the intrafusal fibres [11,18,24] there are a few isolated reports on their presence in these fibres [5,28].

Ultrastructural studies of the rods revealed the following morphological characteristics (page 111) : origin in the Z discs, structural continuity with actin filaments, tetragonal filamentous array in transverse sections, and periodic lines perpendicular and parallel to the long axis of the rods [6,7, 12,13,22].

The composition of the rods is uncertain: actin [7], 6 S-alpha-actinin [27] and 10 S-alpha-actinin [31,32] have been suggested as possible constituents.

Rods are seen in many unrelated neuromuscular disorders. Therefore, their presence in a biopsy cannot be considered as evidence that the patient is suffering from nemaline myopathy.

Although many sporadic cases have been described, in some instances there were indications of an autosomal recessive [24,25] or autosomal dominant [14,16,30] mode of transmission. In a relatively large series of patients, it has been found that there are two types of hereditary nemaline myopathy, which cannot be distinguished from each other on clinical or histological grounds [1]. There is an autosomal recessive type in which both clinically healthy parents may show rods in their biopsies. In addition there is an autosomal dominant type, in which there may be marked variability in clinical expression.

Late onset rod disease

There have been some reports on adult patients with muscular weakness and rods in their muscle biopsies [6,9,10,15,23]. Onset varied from 37 to 60 years of age. In most of these patients the proximal muscles were more involved than the distal muscles. Laboratory findings were variable. In three patients there was an elevation of the ESR. The course was progressive and sometimes led to severe disability [6] or death [9].

In two patients, abundant, highly organized rod-shaped particles were found in the muscle nuclei [9].

References 1 Arts,W.F.,Bethlem,J.,Dingemans,K.P.,Ericsson,A.W.
Investigations on the inheritance of nemaline myopathy.
To be published

2 Badurska,B.,Fidzianska,A.,Jedrzejowska,H.
Nemaline myopathy.
Neuropat.pol.1970,8:389–397

3 Battin,J.,Vital,C.,Vallat,J.-M.,Fontan,D.,LeBlanc,M.
Le myopathie à bâtonnet 'nemaline myopathy'. A propos
d'une observation mortelle. Aspect clinique et ultrastructure.
Sem.Hôp.Paris 1975,51:404–413

4 Conen,P.E.,Murphy,E.G.,Donohue,W.L.
Light and electron microscopic studies of 'myogranules' in
a child with hypotonia and muscle weakness.
Canad.med.Ass.J.1963,89:983–986

5 Dahl,D.S.,Klutzow,F.W.
Congenital rod disease. Further evidence of innervational
abnormalities as the basis for the clinicopathologic feature.
J.neurol.Sci.1974,23:371–385

6 Engel,A.G.
Recent studies on neuromuscular disease. Late-onset
myopathy (a new syndrome?): light and electron
microscopic oservations in two cases.
Proc.Mayo Clin.1966,41:713–741

7 Engel,A.G.,Gomez,M.R.
Nemaline (Z disk) myopathy: observations on the origin,
structure, and solubility properties of the nemaline
structures.
J.Neuropath.exp.Neurol.1967,26:601–619

8 Engel,W.K.,Cunningham,G.C.
Rapid examination of muscle tissue.
Neurology(Minneap.)1963,13:919–923

9 Engel,W.K.,Oberc,M.A.
Abundant nuclear rods in adult-onset rod disease.
J.Neuropath.exp.Neurol.1975,34:119–132

10 Engel,W.K.,Resnick,J.S.
Late-onset rod myopathy: a newly recognized, acquired, and
progressive disease.
Neurology(Minneap.)1966,16:308–309

11 Engel,W.K.,Wanko,T.,Fenichel,G.M.

Nemaline myopathy. A second case.
Arch.Neurol.(Chic.)1964,11:22–39

12   Fardeau,M.
Etude d'une nouvelle observation de 'nemaline myopathy'.
Acta neuropath.1969,13:250–266

13   Gonatas,N.K.
The fine structure of the rod-like bodies in nemaline
myopathy and their relation to the Z-discs.
J.Neuropath.exp.Neurol.1966,25:409–421

14   Gonatas,N.K.,Shy,G.M.,Godfrey,E.H.
Nemaline myopathy. The origin of nemaline structures.
NewEngl.J.Med.1966,274:535–539

15   Heffernan,L.P.,Rewcastle,N.B.,Humphrey,J.G.
The spectrum of rod myopathies.
Arch.Neurol.(Chic.)1968,18:529–542

16   Hopkins,I.J.,Lindsey,J.R.,Ford,F.R.
Nemaline myopathy. A long-term clinicopathologic study of
affected mother and daughter.
Brain 1966,89:299–310

17   Hudgson,P.,Gardner-Medwin,D.,Fulthorpe,J.J.,Walton,J.N.
Nemaline myopathy.
Neurology(Minneap.)1967,17:1125–1142

18   Karpati,G.,Carpenter,S.,Andermann,F.
A new concept of childhood nemaline myopathy.
Arch.Neurol.(Chic.)1971,24:291–304

19   Kuitunen,P.,Rapola,J.,Noponen,A.-L.,Donner,M.
Nemaline myopathy. Report of four cases and review of
the literature.
Acta paediat.scand.1972,61:353–361

20   Kulakowski,S.,Flament-Durand,J.,Malaisse-Lagae,F.,
Chevallay,M.,Fardeau,M.
Myopathie à bâtonnets. ('nemaline myopathy'). Documents
cliniques, histologiques, ultrastructuraux et anatomiques,
concernant une nouvelle observation, d'évolution mortelle
par insuffisance respiratoire.
Arch.franç.Pédiat.1973,30:505–526

21   Lindsey,J.R.,Hopkins,I.J.,Clark,D.B.
Pathology of nemaline myopathy. Studies in two adult cases
including an autopsy.

Bull.Johns Hopk.Hosp.1966,119:378–406

22 McDonald,R.D.,Engel,A.G.
Observations on organization of Z-disk components and
on rod bodies of Z-disk origin.
J.CellBiol.1971,48:431–437

23 Mashiko,N.
A myopathy with abnormal Z-bands.
Neurology(Bombay).1973,20:484–490

24 Neustein,H.B.
Nemaline myopathy. A family study with three autopsied cases.
Arch.Path.1973,96:192–195

25 Nienhuis,A.W.,Coleman,R.F.,Brown,W.J.,Munsat,T.L.,
Pearson,C.M.
Nemaline myopathy. A histopathologic and biochemical
study.
Amer.J.clin.Path.1967,48:1–13

26 Price,H.M.,Gordon,G.B.,Pearson,C.M.,Munsat,T.L.,
Blumberg,J.M.
New Evidence for excessive accumulation of Z-band material
in nemaline myopathy.
Proc.nat.Acad.Sci.USA,1965,54:1398–1406

27 Schollmeyer,J.E.,Goll,D.E.,Robson,R.M.,Stromer,M.H.
Localization of alpha-actinin and tropomyosin in different
muscles.
J.Cell Biol.1973,59:306a

28 Shafiq,S.A.,Dubowitz,V.,Peterson,H.deC.,Milhorat,A.T.
Nemaline myopathy: report of a fatal case, with histochemical
and electron microscopical studies.
Brain 1967,90:817–828

29 Shy,G.M.,Engel,W.K.,Somers,J.E.,Wanko,T.
Nemaline myopathy. A new congenital myopathy.
Brain 1963,86:793–810

30 Spiro,A.J.,Kennedy,C.
Hereditary occurrence of nemaline myopathy.
Arch.Neurol.(Chic.)1965,13:155–159

31 Sugita,H.,Masaki,T.,Ebashi,S.,Pearson,C.M.
Protein composition of rods in nemaline myopathy.
In:Basic Research in Myology.B.A.Kakulas(ed.).
Amsterdam,Excerpta Medica,1973,pp.298–302

32   Sugita,H.,Masaki,T.,Ebashi,S.,Pearson,C.M.
       Staining of nemaline rods by the antibody against
       10S-component of alpha-actinin (10S-actinin).
       In:Abstracts,3rd International Congress on Muscle Diseases.
       Amsterdam,Excerpta Medica,1974,pp.15

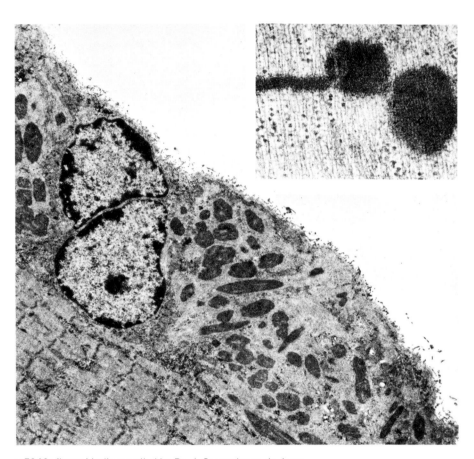

×5040; figure kindly supplied by Dr. J. Stoppelman-de Jong

Inset, ×52,000; figure kindly supplied by Dr. K.P. Dingemans

Rods are small structures, usually about 1–5 μ in length and 0.2–2 μ in diameter, that stain bright red with the modified Gomori trichrome method. They may be present in both fibre types and are devoid of enzyme activity. In and around areas containing rods, vesicular nuclei with prominent nucleoli are frequently present. The electron micrograph shows a collection of rods in the subsarcolemmal region of a muscle fibre. When present in the central area of the fibres, it can be seen that the rods originate from the Z discs, have a structural continuity with actin filaments, and show periodic lines perpendicular and parallel to their long axis (inset). In transverse sections a lattice-like arrangement can be observed.

Rods may be present in the autosomal recessive and dominant types of nemaline myopathy (page 103), in numerous other neuromuscular disorders and in normal muscles, for instance at the myotendinous junctions and in the extra-ocular muscles. Rods have also been observed in muscle fibres displaying other structural changes, such as cores or focal loss of cross-striations.

In 1972, Brooke and Neville [1] described two unrelated young girls who both suffered from a severe myopathy with a fatal outcome.

The patients were born as floppy infants. The motor mile stones were delayed.

One girl showed progressive weakness and wasting of the muscles of the extremities, with profound hypotonia and absent deep tendon reflexes. The serum creatine phosphokinase (CPK) activity was slightly elevated. The electromyogram showed brief, polyphasic motor unit potentials. She died at the age of 9 months from a bilateral pneumonia.

The other girl showed slight bilateral ptosis and facial weakness, with generalized weakness and wasting of the muscles of the extremities, atonia and bilateral contractures of the gastrocnemius, forearm and upper arm muscles. The deep tendon reflexes were depressed. The serum CPK activity was normal. The electromyogram showed short, polyphasic motor unit potentials. Motor nerve conduction velocity was normal. She died at the age of $2\frac{1}{2}$ years from respiratory failure.

Muscle biopsies showed marked variability in the size of the fibres, type I fibre predominance in one case, and a mild degree of fibrosis. Also in both cases a large number of muscle fibres revealed so-called reducing bodies. These bodies were round or oval in shape and were commonly found at the outer edge of the muscle fibres. Single bodies were most commonly seen, but occasional multiple bodies (up to 8 per fibre) were observed. The bodies exhibited reducing activity. They were intensely reactive with the menadione-linked alpha-glycerophosphate dehydrogenase reaction. This was, however, not due to any activity of the enzyme but to the presence of sulphydryl groups. In addition the bodies contained glycogen and ribonucleic acid.

Electron microscopy of the bodies showed that they consisted of closely packed, irregularly shaped and moderately osmiophilic particles, with a diameter of 120–160 Ångströms. Within the matrix of these particles, holes containing glycogen particles, mitochondria, triads and strands of fibrillar material, were present.

A benign congenital myopathy with reducing bodies in 0.2–0.5 per cent of the muscle fibres was described by Tomé and Fardeau [2] in 1975.

The patient was a boy, 14 years of age, with delayed development of motor functions and generalized non-progressive muscular weakness. In addition he had contractures of both gastrocnemii, a high arched palate and pectus carinatus. Serum CPK activity was normal.

Muscle pathology was identical to that of reducing body myopathy, and there was type I predominance. No glycogen, mitochondria or triads were seen within the bodies.

Again, in this case, the reducing activity of the bodies was likely to be due to sulphydryl groups, as was also demonstrated by the positive mercury orange and Chèvremont-Frédéric reactions.

Light and electron microscopy of the motor end-plates and intramuscular nerves did not reveal any abnormalities.

References   1   Brooke,M.H.,Neville,H.E.
                    Reducing body myopathy.
                    Neurology(Minneap.)1972,22:829–840
              2   Tomé,F.M.S.,Fardeau,M.
                    Congenital myopathy with 'reducing bodies' in muscle fibres.
                    Acta neuropath.1975,31:207–217

In 1969, Bethlem, Van Wijngaarden, Meijer and Hülsmann [1] described a 16-year-old girl, born as a floppy infant and with delayed motor development.

Examination revealed marked weakness and atrophy of the flexors of the head, triceps muscles and extensors of the feet and toes. The muscles of the shoulder and pelvic girdles were only slightly involved. The patellar reflexes were present, the other deep tendon reflexes were absent. In addition there was cardiomyopathy of unknown origin.

The serum creatine phosphokinase activity was elevated. Electromyography showed numerous spontaneous fibrillations at rest and motor unit potentials of short duration. The motor nerve conduction velocities were normal. Muscle biopsies revealed type I fibre smallness and central nuclei in about 70 per cent of the type I fibres and about 45 per cent of the type II fibres. Peculiar focal areas (myotube-like structures) were present in the type I fibres. In the transverse sections these consisted of a central granular area, often containing vesicular nuclei, and surrounded by an irregular rim of myofibrils. The central areas showed a high activity of oxidative enzymes and phosphorylase, but no myofibrillar ATPase activity. In longitudinal sections, the abnormal zones occupied only part of the length of the fibres. At both ends a zone of altered myofibrils was seen, at the poles of which short chains of vesicular nuclei extended into the fibre. No ultrastructural studies were made.

The patient's 18-year-old brother suffered from peroneal muscular atrophy from early infancy. The clinically normal father had short-duration motor unit potentials on electromyographic examination and slight atypical histopathological alterations in his muscle biopsy.

Reference   1   Bethlem,J.,VanWijngaarden,G.K.,Meyer,A.E.F.H., Hülsmann,W.C.
Neuromuscular disease with type I fiber atrophy, central nuclei, and myotube-like structures.
Neurology(Minneap.)1969,19:705–710

In 1972, Engel, Angelini and Gomez [2] reported on a congenital non-
progressive myopathy in which abundant abnormal inclusions composed
of complex, convoluted lamellae arranged in fingerprint patterns, were
seen at the ultrastructual level.

The patient was a 5-year-old girl in whom generalized weakness and
hypotonia had been present since infancy. The motor milestones were
delayed. Examination revealed diffuse, moderate weakness of the muscles
of the trunk and extremities. The deep tendon reflexes were decreased
or absent. Intelligence was subnormal, with a normal electroencephalo-
gram. The activity of the serum creatine phosphokinase was normal. The
electromyogram was thought to be consistent with a myopathy. There
were normal motor and sensory nerve conduction velocities.

Histochemical examination of 2 muscle biopsies showed type I fibre predominance, small or normal-sized type I fibres and type II fibre hypertrophy.
In the type I fibres numerous subsarcolemmal inclusions were seen with
phase-optic microscopy. Electron microscopy revealed that these inclusions were composed of concentric lamellae that had a characteristic
spacing and contained sawtooth-shaped sub-units at regular intervals. In
addition, many of the type I fibres showed focal myofibrillar degeneration
associated with a decrease of mitochondria.

Another report concerns two half brothers with a congenital benign myopathy. In their muscle biopsies fingerprint bodies were seen. In both
biopsies there was type I fibre smallness, while in one biopsy type I fibre
predominance was present [3].

This observation of familial incidence of fingerprint body myopathy was
suggestive of a disease entity.

In the muscle biopsy of a 55-year-old woman with a congenital non-
progressive myopathy, fingerprint bodies were also the predominant
morphological abnormality [4].

The occurrence of these bodies in various diseases [6], including other
neuromuscular disorders such as dermatomyositis [1], dystrophia myotonica [6,7] and oculopharyngeal muscular dystrophy [5], indicates that
these formations are a rare but non-specific reaction of the muscle.

References   1   Carpenter,S.,Karpati,G.,Eisen,A.,Andermann,F.,Watters,G.
                      Childhood dermatomyositis and familial collagen disease.
                      Neurology(Minneap.)1972,22:425

                 2   Engel,A.G.,Angelini,M.R.,Gomez,M.R.
                      Fingerprint body myopathy. A newly recognized congenital
                      muscle disease.
                      Proc.Mayo Clin.1972,47:377–388.

                 3   Fardeau,M.,Tomé,F.M.S.,Derambure,S.
                      Familial fingerprint body myopathy.
                      Arch.Neurol.(Chic.)1976,33:724–725

                 4   Gordon,A.S.,Rewcastle,N.B.,Humphrey,J.G.,Stewart,B.M.
                      Chronic benign congenital myopathy: fingerprint body type.
                      Canad.J.neurol.Ass.1974,1:106–113

                 5   Julien,J.,Vital,C.,Vallat,J.M.,Vallat,M.,LeBlanc,M.
                      Oculopharyngeal muscular dystrophy. A case with abnormal
                      mitochondria and 'fingerprint' inclusions.
                      J.neurol.Sci.1974,21:165–169

                 6   Sengel,A.,Stoebner,P.
                      Une inclusion musculaire atypique rare: les 'corps en empreintes
                      digitales' ou 'fingerprint bodies'.
                      Acta neuropath.1974,27:61–68

                 7   Tomé,F.M.S.,Fardeau,M.
                      'Fingerprint inclusions' in muscle fibres in dystrophia
                      myotonica.
                      Acta neuropath.1973,24:62–67

In 1973, Jerusalem, Engel and Gomez [1] reported on a congenital, non-progressive myopathy with segmental vacuolation, especially of type II fibres, due to a pathologic alteration in the sarcotubular system.

The patients were two brothers, 15 en 11 years old, of Russian ancestors and consanguineous parentage. The elder boy had always been awkward in running and had difficulty in climbing stairs. He showed mild weakness of the neck flexors, proximal limb and anterior tibialis muscles. The deep tendon reflexes were normal.

The electromyogram was thought to be consistent with a myopathy. The activity of the serum creatine phosphokinase was increased (360 U/L).

The younger boy was noted to move less in utero than any of the other 9 siblings. He had difficulty in running, climbing stairs and rising from the sitting position.

On examination he showed mild weakness of the facial muscles and moderate weakness of the neck flexors and proximal muscles of all extremities. The deep tendon reflexes were hypoactive, the weak muscles were reduced in bulk. The electromyogram was non-diagnostic. The serum creatine phosphokinase activity was normal. Both patients had normal motor and sensory nerve conduction velocities.

Muscle pathology was characterized by myriad small vacuoles. In transverse sections the vacuoles were dispersed throughout the fibre, but in longitudinal sections the vacuolar change was segmental in distribution. Several segments, ranging from 30 to 150 μ in length, were seen in one fibre. The vacuoles were less than 6 μ wide and reacted negatively for lipids, glycogen, acid mucopolysaccharides and acid phosphatase. Type II fibres were affected more often than type I fibres. Electron microscopy showed that the abnormal spaces were membrane-bound. Electron cytochemical studies indicated that the limiting membranes were reactive for the sarcoplasmic reticulum ATPase. The transverse tubular system retained a close topographic relationship with the abnormal spaces, abutting on their periphery or invaginating into their interior. Morphometric analysis of the electron micrographs indicated that the concentration of non-dilated sarcotubular profiles was significantly increased in the patients' vacuolated fibres above that in normal control fibres. There was no difference between the patients' non-affected fibres and the fibres from the normal control subjects.

Reference   **1**   Jerusalem,F.,Engel,A.G.,Gomez,M.R.
Sarcotubular myopathy. A newly recognized, benign, congenital, familial muscle disease.
Neurology(Minneap.)1973,25:897–906

A congenital myopathy showing rods and zebra bodies (leptomeres) at the ultrastructural level was named zebra body myopathy [1]. These bodies can also be found in normal muscles [2,3] and numerous neuro-muscular diseases.

References   1   Lake,B.D.,Wilson,J.
                          Zebra body myopathy. Clinical, histochemical and
                          ultrastructural studies.
                          J.neurol.Sci.1975,24:437–446
                  2   Mair,W.G.P.,Tomé,F.M.S.
                          Atlas of the Ultrastructure of Diseased Human Muscle.
                          Edinburgh,Livingstone,1972
                  3   Martinez,A.J.,Hay,S.,McNeer,K.W.
                          Extraocular muscles. Light microscopy and ultrastructural
                          features.
                          Acta neuropath.1976,34:237–253

Myopathies with abnormal mitochondria

These myopathies are a collection of heterogeneous neuromuscular diseases which have one thing in common: the presence of a large number of normal, as well as abnormally shaped and enlarged mitochondria in the muscle fibres. In addition, the mitochondria often contain densely packed cristae and paracrystalline inclusions. The latter could be identified as proteins. Light-cored dense particles in the muscle mitochondria were also described [1].

Ultrastructural mitochondrial abnormalities of the muscle fibre can be suspected by light microscopy when there is an accumulation of subsarcolemmal and intermyofibrillar granular material together with an increase of vesicular nuclei.

The granular material stains red with the modified trichrome stain and shows a high activity in sections stained for oxidative enzymes. In addition there may be excessive lipid droplets. Because of the red staining with the modified trichrome method and the irregularity of their internal architectural arrangement and external contours, these fibres were named 'ragged-red fibres' ([4], page 125). In many, but not all cases, this pathological finding is restricted to the type I fibres.

As has been the case in almost all myopathies that were named after one single morphological abnormality, it soon became apparent that the abnormal mitochondrial features were non-specific. Similar changes can be seen in many different unrelated disorders of skeletal muscle (i.e. polymyositis, hypothyroid and thyrotoxic myopathies, spinal muscular atrophy, etc.). Even so, some authors use the name 'mitochondrial myopathy' when − according to their opinion − the mitochondrial abnormality is the most striking morphological finding in the muscle biopsy. This, in spite of the fact that there are other pathological features, for instance, increase of lipid or glycogen. Most authors, however, prefer descriptive names like 'skeletal muscle disease with abnormal mitochondria' [15], 'mitochondria−lipid−glycogen disease of muscle' [9] or 'sudanophilic mitochondrial disease' [6].

In many cases there is also a functional abnormality of the mitochondria, viz. loosely coupled state of oxidative phosphorylation [8]. When mitochondria have retained the ability to oxidize certain substrates, but have lost the ability to phosphorylate adenosine diphosphate (ADP) to adenosine triphosphate (ATP), they are uncoupled. When the rate of respiration of mitochondria in the presence of inorganic phosphate cannot be increased by adding ADP, but these particles can still couple respiration to phosphorylation of ADP to ATP, this state of respiration is defined as loosely coupled. This functional abnormality can be found in many unrelated neuromuscular disorders [5] and is non-specific. Therefore, the loosely coupled state of oxidative phosphorylation of the muscle mitochondria is considered to be a secondary phenomenon of various unknown metabolic abnormalities, and is not the primary cause of the symptomatology.

Difficulties in classification have been increased by the fact that some authors put forward another feature that is often encountered in this group of myopathies, namely chronic lactic acidosis [7,13,14].
The importance of the increased blood lactate level — no doubt also a secondary phenomenon — was stressed by describing the disorder as "chronic lactic acidosis in association with myopathy" [14].
A severe hypermetabolic state with systemic lactic acidosis and the presence of ragged-red fibres, was produced in rats by infusion of uncouplers of mitochondrial oxidative phosphorylation [10].

All kinds of sporadic, familial and hereditary myopathies with abnormal mitochondria have been described. Clinically, there may be generalized, limb-girdle [2], facioscapulohumeral (page 136) or distal (page 52) muscular involvement. Onset is at all ages, from birth [12] or early childhood [3,8,12] till the end of the fifth decade [11].
In addition to the muscular weakness many other manifestations can be observed: severe hypermetabolism of non-thyroid origin (page 128), salt craving (page 131), excessive fatigability (page 133), growth retardation [3,7,14], nerve eafness [7] and the many features of oculocraniosomatic neuromuscular disease (page 63).

References   1   Bender,A.N.,Engel,W.K.
Light-cored dense particles in mitochondria of a patient
with skeletal muscle and myocardial disease.
J.Neuropath.exp.Neurol.1976,35:46–52

2   Black,J.T.,Judge,D.,Demers,L.,Gordon,S.
Ragged-red fibers. A biochemical and morphological study.
J.neurol.Sci.1975,26:479–488

3   D'Agostino,A.N.,Ziter,F.A.,Rallison,M.L.,Bray,P.F.
Familial myopathy with abnormal muscle mitochondria.
Arch.Neurol.(Chic.).1968,18:388–401

4   Engel,W.K.
'Ragged-red fibers' in ophthalmoplegia syndromes and
their differential diagnosis.
In:Abstracts of the 2nd International Congress on
Muscle Diseases,Perth,November 22–26,1971.
Amsterdam,Excerpta Medica,1971,p.28.(Int.Congr.Ser.237).

5   Gimeno,A.,Trueba,J.L.,Blanco,M.,Gosalvez,M.
Mitochondrial functions in five cases of human neuromuscular
disorders.
J.Neurol.Neurosurg.Psychiat.1973,36:806–812

6   Gullotta,F.,Payk,T.R.,Solbach,A.
Sudanophile (mitochondriale) Myopathie.
Z.Neurol.1974,206:309–326

7   HackettJr,T.N.,Bray,P.F.,Ziter,F.A.,Nyhan,W.L.,Creer,K.M.
A metabolic myopathy associated with chronic lactic acidemia,
growth failure, and nerve deafness.
J.Pediat.1973,83:426–431

8   Hülsmann,W.C.,Bethlem,J.,Meijer,A.E.F.H.,Fleury,P.,
Schellens,J.P.M.
Myopathy with abnormal structure and function of muscle
mitochondria.
J.Neurol.Neurosurg.Psychiat.1967,30:519–525

9   Jerusalem,F.,Angelini,C.,Engel,A.G.,Groover,R.V.
Mitochondria-lipid-glycogen (MLG) disease of muscle.
A morphologically regressive congenital myopathy.
Arch.Neurol.(Chic.)1973,29:162–169

10   Melmed,C.,Karpati,G.,Carpenter,S.
Experimental mitochondrial myopathy produced by in vivo
uncoupling of oxidative phosphorylation.
J.neurol.Sci.1975,26:305–318

11 Shibasaki,H.,Santa,T.,Kuroiwa,Y.
Late onset mitochondrial myopathy.
J.neurol.Sci.1973,18: 301–310

12 Shy,G.M.,Gonatas,N.K.,Perez,M.
Two childhood myopathies with abnormal mitochondria.
I. Megaconial myopathy. II. Pleoconial myopathy.
Brain 1966,89:133–158

13 Sluga,E.,Monneron,A.
Ueber die Feinstruktur und Topochemie von
Riesenmitochondrien und deren Einlagerungen bei
Myopathien.
Virchows Arch.Abt.A.Path.Anat.1970,350:250–260

14 Tarlow,M.J.,Lake,B.D.,Lloyd,J.K.
Chronic lactic acidosis in association with myopathy.
Arch.Dis.Childh. 1973,48:489–492

15 Van Wijngaarden,G.K.,Bethlem,J.,Meijer,A.E.F.H.,
Hülsmann,W.C.,Feltkamp,C.A.
Skeletal muscle disease with abnormal mitochondria.
Brain 1967,90:577–592

Ragged-red fibres show large collections of normal, as well as abnormally shaped and enlarged mitochondria.

With light microscopy these mitochondria can be recognized as, mainly subsarcolemmal, accumulations of granules. These stain bright red with the modified Gomori trichrome stain and show excessive oxidative enzyme activities. In these areas, an increase of glycogen and lipid may be present, while there is frequently a proliferation of vesicular nuclei with prominent nucleoli.

The contours of the fibres are irregular, hence the name ragged-red fibres. Section A (page 126), stained for NADH-tetrazolium reductase activity, shows ragged-red fibres with a very high enzyme activity in the subsarcolemmal regions. All affected fibres are type I fibres.

In B (page 126) there are three ragged-red fibres, with irregular external contours and an abnormal coarse distribution of the oxidative enzyme activity.

In C (page 127) a collection of enlarged and bizarrely shaped mitochondria is seen. The inset shows a large mitochondrion with paracrystalline inclusions.

Ragged-red fibres may be abundantly present in the various myopathies with abnormal mitochondria (page 121) and in oculocraniosomatic neuromuscular disease (page 63).

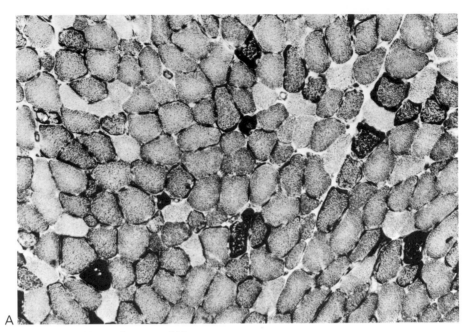

NADH-tetrazolium reductase, ×110

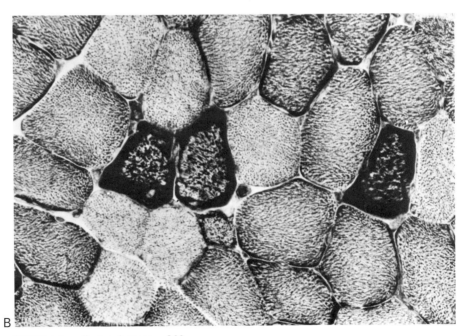

NADH-tetrazolium reductase, ×260

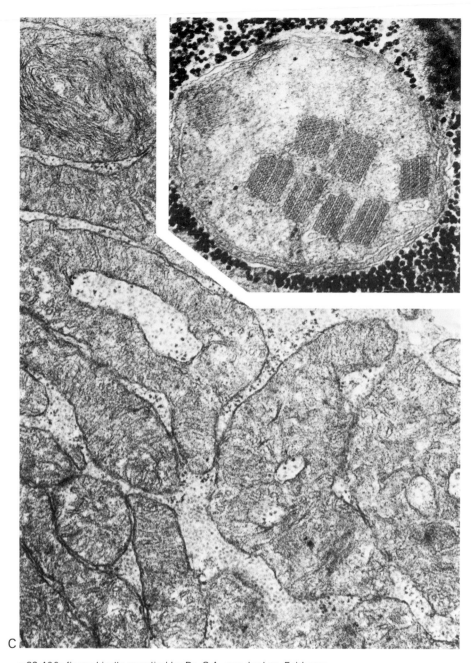

×32,400; figure kindly supplied by Dr. C.A. van der Lee-Feltkamp

Inset, ×48,600; figure kindly supplied by Dr. J. Stoppelman-de Jong

In 1962 Luft, Ikkos, Palmieri, Ernster and Afzelius [6] gave the first detailed description of a patient suffering from a myopathy with abnormal mitochondria and severe hypermetabolism. Other reports on the biochemical properties of the muscle mitochondria in this patient were published by the same group [3,4]. The patient was a female in whom the first signs became apparent in early childhood, when she began to complain of increased perspiration, chiefly at night. This became more marked at the age of 7 years and persisted into adult life with little change. Apart from continuous and severe perspiration, she suffered from polydipsia, polyphagia, marked underweight, raised skin temperature and progressive asthenia.

Examination revealed muscular weakness, poorly developed muscles, hypotonia and hyperflexibility. The tendon reflexes were absent. There was creatinuria. The electromyogram showed short and polyphasic action potentials.

A striking feature was severe hypermetabolism with a basal metabolic rate usually between +140 and +210 per cent. The thyroid function was normal while none of the known extrathyroidal causes of hypermetabolism could be demonstrated.

Light-microscopic investigation of a muscle biopsy showed subcarcolemmal zones, sometimes filled with granules.

Electron microscopy revealed in the subsarcolemmal parts of the muscle fibres an increased number of abnormal mitochondria of variable shape and size. Many mitochondria showed densely packed cristae and tubular internal structures.

No morphological abnormalities were seen in the mitochondria of the skin and the uterine mucosa. Biochemical studies of mitochondria isolated from the muscle tissue, revealed a loosely coupled state of oxidative phosphorylation.

Another case with similar clinical and pathological features was published ten years later [1]. This 19-year-old female showed modest generalized muscle weakness without wasting and with normal tendon reflexes. Intolerance to heat was so severe that she slept in a tub of cold water during the summer.

The BMR ranged from +200 to +300 per cent.

Serum creatine phosphokinase activity was normal. A state of loosely coupled oxidative phosphorylation of the isolated muscle mitochondria was also present [2,5]. The ultrastructural features of a biopsy of the skin, intestine and liver were normal. Because of its depressant effect on protein synthesis in mitochondria, chloramphenicol was tried experimentally in this patient. Treatment with this drug resulted in a significant decrease in BMR, associated with improvement in the clinical picture.

Exhaustive biochemical studies were made in the same patient [2]. At that time she showed mild weakness of the psoas muscles, but none elsewhere, while no effect was seen by administration of chloramphenicol. The rate of calcium uptake by the isolated muscle mitochondria was normal, but the total amount of calcium taken up, was much decreased. The accumulated calcium could not be retained and was spontaneously released, suggesting that recycling of calcium could take place in vivo and result in sustained stimulation of respiration and loose coupling.

References   1   Afifi,A.K.,Ibrahim,M.Z.M.,Bergman,R.A.,Haydar,N.A.,
                            Mire,J.,Bahuth,N.,Kaylani,F.
                            Morphologic features of hypermetabolic mitochondrial
                            disease. A light microscopic, histochemical and electron
                            microscopic study.
                            J.neurol.Sci.1972,15:271–290
                    2   DiMauro,S.,Bonilla,E.,Lee,C.P.,Schotland,D.L.,Scarpa,A.,
                            ConnJr,H.,Chance,B.
                            Luft's disease. Further biochemical and ultrastructural studies
                            of skeletal muscle in the second case.
                            J.neurol.Sci.1976,27:217–232
                    3   Ernster,L.,Ikkos,D.,Luft,R.
                            Enzymatic activities of human skeletal muscle mitochondria:
                            a tool in clinical metabolic research.
                            Nature(Lond.)1959,184:1851–1854
                    4   Ernster,L.,Luft,R.
                            Further studies on a population of human skeletal muscle
                            mitochondria lacking respiratory control.
                            Exp.Cell Res.1963,32:26–35

5   Haydar,N.A.,Conn,H.L.,Afifi,A.,Wakid,N.,Ballas,S.,Fawaz,K.
Severe hypermetabolism with primary abnormality of skeletal
muscle mitochondria.
Ann.intern.Med.1971,74:548–558

6   Luft,R.,Ikkos,D.,Palmieri,G.,Ernster,L.,Afzelius,B.
A case of severe hypermetabolism of nonthyroid origin with
a defect in the maintenance of mitochondrial respiratory
control: a correlated clinical, biochemical, and morphologic
study.
J.clin.Invest.1962,41:1776–1804

The association of a limb-girdle myopathy with severe craving for salt was described in 1966 by Shy, Gonatas and Perez [2] in one of the first papers on myopathies with abnormal mitochondria. This disease was then called 'pleoconial myopathy' because of the abundance of moderately enlarged mitochondria.

The patient was a 8-year-old boy who was floppy at birth. The motor milestones were delayed. On examination he showed a non-progressive severe proximal and moderate distal muscle weakness. The deep tendon reflexes were hypoactive. Blood and urine analysis were all within normal limits.

Electromyographical findings were consistent with a myopathy. The motor nerve conduction velocities were normal.

In addition he suffered from episodes of increasing muscular weakness with severe quadriparesis, each occurring at night and noted in the morning when he awakened. He was then unable to move, his speech became indistinct, he became nauseated, vomited and perspired profusely. During these periods he had a severe craving for salt, which he ingested by the teaspoon. These periods lasted one or two weeks. Less severe attacks of increasing muscle weakness in the morning occurred once or twice a week and lasted several hours. No attacks of muscle weakness could be elicited by vigorous exercise, restriction of sodium intake, potassium loading or with aldosterone antagonists.

A muscle biopsy showed subsarcolemmal and intermyofibrillar granules, staining purple-red with the modified trichrome stain and showing high oxidative enzyme activity. Ultrastructural studies revealed large areas of densely packed mitochondria that were tremendously increased in number. The 12-year-old sister of the patient also suffered from excessive salt craving.

A patient with similar clinical signs and symptoms was described in 1970 by Spiro, Prineas and Moore [3]. This 13-year-old boy had on one occasion an episode of increased generalized muscle weakness lasting 2–3 hours. Marked craving for salt had been present all his life. Ischaemic forearm exercise was followed by a normal rise in the blood lactate level.

Muscle biopsy showed no fibre type differentiation and there was an increase in staining for lipid and oxidative enzymatic activity. Electron microscopy revealed a marked increase of mitochondria, somewhat larger and more irregular in shape than usual. Isolated mitochondria revealed a state of loose coupling of oxidative phosphorylation.

In this patient there was no family history of neuromuscular disease.

In sodium-responsive, normokalaemic periodic paralysis, described by Poskanzer and Kerr [1], there is often a history of high salt intake. Although these patients also have episodes in which they awaken with severe generalized muscle weakness, they show no hypotonia at birth, and the muscle pathology differs from the cases described above. Moreover, there is an autosomal dominant inheritance.

References   1   Poskanzer,D.C.,Kerr,D.N.S.
                        A third type of periodic paralysis, with normokalemia and
                        favourable response to sodium chloride.
                        Amer.J.Med.1961,31:328–342
              2   Shy,G.M.,Gonatas,N.K.,Perez,M.
                        Two childhood myopathies with abnormal mitochondria.
                        I. Megaconial myopathy. II. Pleoconial myopathy.
                        Brain 1966,89:133–158
              3   Spiro,A.J.,Prineas,J.W.,Moore,C.L.
                        A new mitochondrial myopathy in a patient with salt craving.
                        Arch.Neurol.(Chic.)1970,22:259–269

In 1967, Price, Gordon, Munsat and Pearson [5] described a 20-year-old male who had experienced easy fatigability after muscular exercise from the age of 8 years. This symptom progressed, so that with less exertion he experienced greater fatigue. The fatigue was relieved by a 5– to 10-minute period of rest. There had been no muscle pain or pigmenturia.

Examination revealed mild proximal muscle weakness. He also had signs of a right brachial plexus injury, present since birth. The tendon reflexes were decreased.

Serum creatine phosphokinase activity was normal. There was only a very slight or no rise of serum lactate after ischaemic forearm exercise.

The electromyogram revealed diffuse but mild myopathic changes. Nerve conduction velocities were within normal limits.

Muscle biopsy showed an increase in the number of mitochondria and the presence of many abnormal mitochondria containing paracrystalline inclusions.

In addition, this was associated with an increased number of intracellular deposits of lipid. These abnormalities were restricted to the type I fibres.

A second patient [7] was also a 20-year-old male who noticed unusual fatigability from the age of 8 years. This tendency progressed so much that at the age of 12 years sustained normal physical activity – for instance cycling – became impossible. On his way to school his tiredness was so evident that he was forced to get off his bicycle and to lay down near the road side.

Examination showed no neurological abnormalities. The heart was slightly enlarged and a systolic murmur was heard. At the age of 19 years he started to complain of pain in his limb muscles during exertion.

Serum creatine phospholinase activity was normal. There was an elevated level of venous lactate at rest, with a slight rise after ischaemic forearm exercise. Mitochondrial abnormalities were restricted to the type I fibres.

The isolated muscle mitochondria showed a loosely coupled state of oxidative phosphorylation. At the age of 21 years the patient developed a generalized muscle weakness, more pronounced in the lower legs [4]. Electromyography at that time disclosed signs of denervation in the muscles of the legs, with normal motor conduction velocity of the right peroneal nerve. In addition, there were sensory disturbances in the legs. A few months afterwards the patient died. Post-mortem studies showed cardiomegaly and denervation atrophy in the muscles of the legs, in addition to the abnormalities already found in the biopsy.

Although excessive fatigability on exercise was the prominent symptom in the two patients reported above, this complaint was also a striking feature in some other patients with abnormal muscle mitochondria. These patients showed generalized weakness [1,2], congenital cataract and cardiomyopathy [8] or oculocraniosomatic neuromuscular disease [3].
It may well be that, in some cases, abnormal fatigue can persist for many years, and is subsequently followed by other neuromuscular and somatic symptoms. This is also illustrated by the observation of a 19-year-old boy [6] who suffered from fatigue on exertion for 7 years before he developed muscular weakness.

References   1   Coleman,R.F.,Nienhuis,A.W.,Brown,W.J.,Munsat,T.L., Pearson,C.M.
New myopathy with mitochondrial enzyme hyperactivity. Histochemical demonstration.
J.Amer.med.Ass.1967,199:624–630

2   D'Agostino,A.N.,Ziter,F.A.,Rallison,M.L.,Bray,P.F.
Familial myopathy with abnormal muscle mitochondria.
Arch.Neurol.(Chic.)1968,18:388–401

3   Morgan-Hughes,J.A.,Mair,W.G.P.
Atypical muscle mitochondria in oculoskeletal myopathy.
Brain 1973,96:215–224

4   Ossentjuk,E.
Personal communication.

5   Price,H.M.,Gordon,G.B.,Munsat,T.L.,Pearson,C.M.
Myopathy with atypical mitochondria in type I skeletal muscle fibers. A histochemical and ultrastructural study.
J.Neuropath.exp.Neurol.1967,26:475–497

6 Rawles,J.M.,Weller,R.O.
Familial association of metabolic myopathy, lactic acidosis
and sideroblastic anemia.
Amer.J.Med.1974,56:891–897

7 Schellens,J.P.M.,Ossentjuk,E.
Mitochondrial ultrastructure with crystalloid inclusions in an
unusual type of human myopathy.
Virchows Arch.Abt.B.Zellpath.1969,4:21–29

8 Sengers,R.C.A.,TerHaar,B.G.A.,Trijbels,J.M.F.,Willems,J.L.,
Daniels,O.,Stadhouders,A.M.
Congenital cataract and mitochondrial myopathy of skeletal
and heart muscle associated with lactic acidosis after exercise.
J.Pediat.1975,86:873–880

In 1972 Hudgson, Bradley and Jenkison [1] described a familial slowly progressive myopathy, characterized by a facioscapulohumeral distribution of the muscle weakness and the presence of large numbers of abnormal mitochondria with paracrystalline inclusions. The authors concluded that the mitochondrial abnormality was primary, and consequently named the disease familial 'mitochondrial' myopathy.

Six siblings suffered from this disease. In one patient the muscular weakness was confined to the limb-girdles, without involvement of the face. External ocular movements were normal in all patients. The age at onset ranged widely from 6 to 50 years, the duration ranged from 6 to 19 years, but none of the patients had become confined to a wheel-chair. The serum creatine phosphokinase activity was slightly raised in half the cases.
The electromyogram was consistent with a myopathy. Motor nerve conduction velocities were normal.
In a muscle biopsy of the propositus and of one clinically unaffected sibling with a raised serum creatine phosphokinase activity, areas with coarse granules and vesicular nuclei were present. Both type I and type II fibres were involved and showed a high oxidative enzyme activity and, less commonly, an excessive amount of lipid in the Oil red O stained sections. Electron microscopy revealed an increase of mitochondria, often of bizarre shape, with various abnormalities of cristae, and paracrystalline ('parking lot') inclusions. Isolated muscle mitochondria demonstrated a loosely coupled state of oxidative phosphorylation. In addition, there was an excess of lipid, mainly triglyceride, in the muscle tissue [2].
In this family there was an autosomal dominant mode of inheritance. It was observed that transmission always took place via the maternal line.

References 1 Hudgson,P.,Bradley,W.G.,Jenkison,M.
Familial 'mitochondrial' myopathy. A myopathy associated with disordered oxidative metabolism in muscle fibres.
Part 1. Clinical, electrophysiological and pathological findings.
J.Neurol.Sci.1972,16:343–370

2   Worsfold,M.,Park,D.C.,Pennington,R.J.
     Familial 'mitochondrial' myopathy. A myopathy associated
     with disordered oxidative metabolism in muscle fibres.
     Part 2. Biochemical findings.
     J.neurol.Sci.1973,19: 261—274

In 1970, Spiro, Moore, Prineas, Strasberg and Rapin [2] reported on a father and son, both suffering from an unusual disease of the muscles and of the nervous system.

The father, aged 46 years, had a history of unsteadiness and slurred speech from the age of 33 years. He subsequently suffered from progressive weakness of the muscles of his legs and shoulders and also experienced painful muscle cramps; the latter subsided spontaneously after approximately six years. From the age of about 49 years there was a slight memory deterioration.

Examination revealed proximal weakness of the muscles of the arms and legs, with fasciculations, absent tendon reflexes and extensor plantar reponses. His gait was moderately ataxic. Except for slightly dimished proprioception in the legs, there were no sensory disturbances.

The serum creatine phosphokinase activity was increased.

The electromyogram, which was consistent with a neuropathic process, revealed fibrillations at rest and single motor unit potentials of long duration. Motor nerve conduction velocities were decreased.

His 16-year-old son showed bilateral ptosis, limitation of convergence, predominantly proximal weakness, and bilateral foot drop. In addition there were extensor plantar responses, absent tendon reflexes, cerebellar symptoms, impaired proprioception in the legs, chorioretinitis, intracranial calcifications and myoclonic jerks.

Electromyography and motor nerve conduction velocities were normal.

Muscle biopsies in both patients showed pathological features of concomitant neurogenic atrophy and non-specific myopathy.

Electron microscopy revealed an increase in the number, and a slight increase in the size, of the mitochondria, but the shape and structure were normal. Studies on the isolated muscle mitochondria showed a marked reduction in the cytochrome b content, an abnormal insensitivity to antimycin A and a loosely coupled state of oxidative phosphorylation.

The exact relationship between the clinical, morphological and biochemical findings remained uncertain.

Observation of another patient revealed progressive predominant proximal weakness. There was also a marked and progressive increase in muscle weakness during substained contraction or repetitive muscular exercise. The muscle biopsy showed ragged-red fibres (page 125). In vitro studies of isolated muscle mitochondria revealed a loosely coupled state of oxidative phosphorylation and deficiency of reducable cytochrome b [1].

References   1   Morgan-Hughes,J.A.,Clark,J.
                    Mitochondrial myopathy characterized by cytochrome-B
                    deficiency.
                    Paper read at the Oxford Symposium on Muscle Diseases,
                    Oxford,9–10 July,1976
                 2   Spiro,A.J.,Moore,C.L.,Prineas,J.W.,Strasberg,P.M.,Rapin,I.
                    A cytochrome-related inherited disorder of the nervous system
                    and muscle.
                    Arch.Neurol.(Chic.)1970,23:103–112

Myotonic disorders

The myotonic disorders consist of a group of non-related, usually hereditary diseases, having in common the presence of clinical myotonia. This is the phenomenon of a failure of the muscle to relax immediately after cessation of voluntary muscular contraction. It is best seen when the patient is asked to release the tightly clenched fist. It can also be seen in the orbicularis oculi muscles when the patient tries to open the firmly closed eyes. Myotonia of the eyelids (myotonic lid lag) can be provoked when the patient is asked to look down following prior sustained upward gaze. The upper eyelids then remain hung up for 10–20 seconds.

The symptom myotonia is described by the patient as stiffness or cramp of the muscles but is never accompanied by pain.

Repetition of muscular contraction can eliminate or improve myotonia, but sometimes it increases its severity (myotonia paradoxa). It is often aggravated by exposure to cold.

Myotonia can also be elicited by percussion of the muscle, for instance with a reflex hammer. This mechanical myotonia presents as a dimple that persists for several seconds. It can usually be demonstrated in the thenar eminences, the tongue, the extensor muscles of the forearms and in the calves.

In the myotonic disorders, electromyography shows high-frequency repetitive discharges that first increase in frequency and amplitude and then rapidly diminish. The myotonic discharges may be evoked by percussion of the muscle, by volitional activity or by movement of the needle-electrode. In the loud-speaker they produce a sound that has been compared with the noise of a dive-bomber.

Electromyographic myotonia, without clinical myotonia, may be present in acid maltase deficiency and denervation.

Myotonia is of muscular origin and does not depend on motor nerve activity, as is indicated by its persistence following curarization or after blocking the motor nerve.

The following diseases in which clinical myotonia is present, are recognized:

Dystrophia myotonica or myotonic dystrophy, myotonia atrophica, Steinert's disease or Steinert-Curschmann's disease (page 147).

Myotonia congenita. There is an autosomal dominant type also called Thomsen's disease and an autosomal recessive type, first described by Becker (page 162).

Familial hyperkalaemic periodic paralysis or paramyotonica congenita (Eulenburg) or adynamia episodica hereditaria (pages 175 and 176).

Familial hypokalaemic periodic paralysis (page 172).

Paralysis periodica paramyotonica described by Becker [1]. This autosomal dominantly inherited disease is considered to be an condition distinct from familial hyperkalaemic periodic paralysis [2]. Myotonia is a prominent feature, and is also present when the patient is exposed to a warm environment. The paralytic attacks are independent of exposure to cold. The muscular weakness is mainly present in the lower extremities. The attacks occur at night, their frequency is low and the duration long. They can be provoked by ingestion of potassium.

Chondrodystrophic myotonia or osteo-chondro-muscular dystrophy, or Schwartz-Jampel syndrome (page 164).

Myopathia myotonica. A non-progressive disease with autosomal dominant inheritance described by Stöhr, Schlote, Bundschu and Reichenmiller [15]. Action myotonia was present in the orbicularis oculi muscles only, while no percussion myotonia was observed. Electromyography, however, showed myotonic discharges in many muscles. In addition, repetitive contraction of the muscles resulted in marked painful contracture and weakness of the exercised muscles. This phenomenon was restricted to the upper extremities.

Myotonia levior. A disease with autosomal dominant inheritance, described by De Jong [4]. The patients have almost no complaints and show only slight myotonia, mainly after percussion of the tongue.

Myotonia and increased muscle irritability. A disease with autosomal dominant inheritance associated with muscular hypertrophy, described by Torbergsen [16] and thought to be a disorder distinct from Thomsen's disease.

Myotonia with myokymia, hyperhydrosis and muscle wasting is a syndrome mainly seen in young adult males. The disorder runs a benign course of variable duration. Although active and percussion myotonia were present in some of the patients [5,6] these features are often lacking.
Another possible similar syndrome was reported by Isaacs [7,–9] under the clinical-descriptive name 'continuous muscle fibre activity'. These patients showed marked generalized muscle stiffness, mainly distal weakness, fasciculations and persistent sweating. There was spontaneous gradual improvement and complete recovery in most cases. The syndrome was thought to be a defect at the level of the terminal fibres of the lower motor neuron. Electron miscroscopy showed hypertrophy and ramification of the secondary synaptic clefts [14].
Although the patients find it difficult to relax their muscles and the stiffness may improve with repeated motions, no dimple is seen after percussion of the muscle. There are also electromyographical distinctions between this phenomenon (also called neuromyotonia [11]) and true myotonia [8,17]. Electromyography shows continuous high-voltage electrical activity at rest. Moreover, in contrast to myotonia, the spontaneous activity in the syndrome of continuous muscle fibre activity is blocked by curare.
The muscle stiffness can be reduced dramatically by treatment with diphenylhydantoin and carbamazepine [7,11,17,18].

Myotonia, with muscular hypertrophy and weakness that can be corrected by exercise is a syndrome described in the French literature [3,12,13].

The onset of the symptoms may be in early childhood. The patients complain of weakness of the muscles after rest. While in bed in the morning, the patients find it difficult to get up. Also, climbing stairs may be difficult, especially the first steps. This weakness disappears after exercise ('warming-up') of the musculature during several minutes.

On examination, there is hypertrophy of the muscles, mainly involving the proximal muscles of the extremities. Slight atrophy of the sternomastoids and facial muscles [13] and the anterior compartment muscles of the legs [3] were also observed. All tendon reflexes, except the biceps reflexes, were found to be absent in one case [13].

Widespread percussion myotonia and electromyographic myotonia were present in all cases, while myotonia after making a fist was also found [12]. Exposure to cold may aggravate the initial muscular weakness and the myotonia [3], but had no influence in most cases.

Muscle biopsies were normal [3,13] or showed atrophy of type II fibres [3,12] and hypertrophy of type I fibres.

Familial occurrence (brother and sister) was observed in a patient with consanguineous parents [12].

References 1 Becker,P.E.
Paramyotonia congenita (Eulenburg).
Stuttgart,Thieme,1970.(Fortschritte der allgemeinen und klinischen Humangenetik;Bd.III)

2 Becker,P.E.
Genetic approaches to the nosology of muscle disease: myotonias and similar diseases.
Birth Def.,Orig.Art.Ser.1971,7:52–62

3 Castaigne,P.,Laplane,D.,Augustin,P.,Dordain,G.,Penders,C.
Myotonie congénitale, faiblesse musculaire corrigée par l'exercise et hypertrophie musculaire.
Rev.Neurol.1973,129:52–57

4 DeJong,J.G.Y.
Myotonia levior.
In:Symposium über progressive Muskeldystrophie.
E.Kuhn(ed.).Berlin,Springer,1966,pp.255–259

5 Gamstorp,I.,Wohlfart,G.
   A syndrome characterized by myokymia, myotonia, muscular
   wasting and increased perspiration.
   Acta psychiat.scand.1959,34:181–194
6 Greenhouse,A.H.,Bicknell,J.M.,Pesch,R.N.,Seelinger,D.F.
   Myotonia, myokymia, hyperhidrosis, and wasting of muscle.
   Neurology(Minneap.)1967,17:263–268
7 Isaacs,H.
   A syndrome of continuous muscle-fibre activity.
   J.Neurol.Neurosurg.Psychiat.1961,24:319–325
8 Isaacs,H.
   Continuous muscle fibre activity in an Indian male with
   additional evidence of terminal motor fibre abnormality.
   J.Neurol.Neurosurg.Psychiat.1967,30:126–133
9 Isaacs,H.,Heffron,J.J.A.
   The syndrome of 'continuous muscle-fibre activity' cured:
   further studies.
   J.Neurol.Neurosurg.Psychiat.1974,37:1231–1235
10 Kuhn,E.,Seiler,D.
   Biochemische Besonderheiten und Unterschiede der
   autosomal dominant und autosomal recessiv vererbten
   Myotonia congenita.
   Klin.Wschr.1970,48:1134–1136
11 Mertens,H.-G.,Zschocke,S.
   Neuromyotonie.
   Klin.Wschr.1965,43:917–925
12 Pépin,B.,Haguenau,M.,Mikol,J.
   Observation familiale de myotonie avec hypertrophie
   musculaire, faiblesse corrigée par l'effort et atrophie des
   fibres de type II.
   Rev.Neurol.1975,131:285–292
13 Sabouraud,O.,Bourel,M.,Chatel,M.,LeBars,J.
   Faiblesse musculaire corrigée par l'exercise accompagnant
   une hypertrophie musculaire avec myotonie.
   Rev.Neurol.1965,112:546–549
14 Sroka,H.,Bornstein,B.,Sandbank,U.
   Ultrastructure of the syndrome of continuous muscle fibre
   activity.
   Acta neuropath.1975,31:85–90

15 Stöhr,M.,Schlote,W.,Bundschu,H.D.,Reichenmiller,H.
Myopathia myotonica. Fallbericht über eine neuartige
hereditäre metabolische Myopathie.
J.Neurol.1975,210:41–66

16 Torbergsen,T.
A family with dominant hereditary myotonia, muscular
hypertrophy, and increased muscular irritability, distinct
from myotonia congenita Thomsen.
Acta neurol.scand.1975,51:225–232

17 Wallis,W.E.,VanPosnak,A.,Plum,F.
Generalized muscular stiffness, fasciculations, and myokymia
of peripheral nerve origin.
Arch.Neurol.(Chic.)1970,22:430–439

18 Welch,L.K.,Appenzeller,O.,Bicknell,J.M.
Peripheral neuropathy with myokymia, sustained muscular
contraction, and continuous motor unit activity.
Neurology(Minneap.)1972,22:161–169

Dystrophia myotonica or myotonic dystrophy is also named Steinert's disease, after the author who, in 1909, gave a full and detailed — though not the first — description of this disease. After Curschmann had suggested using the name dystrophia myotonica instead of myotonia atrophica, it was also called Steinert-Curschmann's disease, especially by German authors. To-day, the name myotonia atrophica has again been put forward, because the muscular features are thought to be due to chronic lower motor neuron involvement [23].

Age of onset

The first symptoms usually start between the ages of 15 and 35 years. A specific clinical syndrome may be present at birth (neonatal dystrophia myotonica, page 153). Many patients have few or no complaints. Therefore, the age of onset is difficult to assess and is probably lower than generally accepted. The majority of the patients who show evident signs of the disease die before the age of 50 years.

Muscular manifestations

Myotonia (page 141) often precedes the symptoms of muscular weakness. It is especially seen when the patient is asked to release the tightly clenched fist.

Percussion myotonia may be present in many muscles, but usually can be best demonstrated in the thenar eminence, the tongue, the extensor muscles of the forearm and in the calves.

Finally, myotonic discharges can be seen during electromyography.

As a rule, myotonia is not a dominating feature in patients suffering from dystrophia myotonica. As it seldom gives rise to disablement, treatment of the myotonia is generally not indicated or even necessary [66].

Ptosis, facial weakness and atrophy of the temporalis and masseter muscles give the patient a characteristic appearance. In addition there is progressive weakness and wasting of the sternomastoids, the muscles of the back and the abdomen, the forearms, the hands and the anterior compartment of the lower legs. Involvement of the musculature of the shoulder and pelvic girdles is less pronounced. Diminished peristaltic amplitude in the pharynx, in the upper part as well as in the smooth muscle portion of the lower part of the oesophagus, was demonstrated by intraluminal mano-metric studies [62]. Poor peristalsis and marked dilatation of the oeso-phagus was seen by contrast cineradiography [28].

Disfunction of the smooth muscles of other organs plays no significant role, although sprue-like disturbances may occur.

The tendon reflexes are reduced or absent, especially in the upper extrem-ities. There is often no relationship between the areflexia and the severity of muscle involvement.

Cataract
Cataract may be present in the first decade, but is usually found between the ages of 25–50 years. When looked for by slit lamp examination, it may be observed in over 90 per cent of the adult patients [39]. White or coloured fine opacities are seen, mainly in the subcapsular part of the posterior cortex. This typical cataract may be the only sign of the disease [10,66].

Retinal alterations
Peripheral fine pigmentations have been observed in a number of pa-tients [4]. Electroretinographic records showed a decrease of the ampli-tude of the b wave [63].

Involvement of the endocrine glands
Fairly constant findings are atrophy of the testes and menstruation distur-bances [7]. Less frequently, reduced thyroid function [42] and atoxic struma [66] are present. The association with hyperthyroidism is very rare [48]. There is a normal thyrotropin-releasing hormone response [59]. Marked increase of the symptoms of myotonia and muscular weakness during pregnancy, with definite improvement within two weeks of delivery, have been described [8].

Abnormalities in glucose tolerance (flat or diabetic curves) have been noted by many authors. The incidence and degree of a biphasic response was found to be significantly increased [58]. A markedly exaggerated plasma insulin response to oral glucose administration may be found in patients [18,29,37] and their clinically unaffected relatives [51,68].

Frontoparietal alopecia

This baldness is frequently noted in the males. It may already be present in the beginning of the second decade. There seems to be no relationship with gonadal atrophy.

Radiological changes in the skull

These are often present [13] and consist of diffuse hyperostosis, hyperostosis frontalis interna [10,12], a small sella turcica [10,12,69], ossification of the diaphragma sella [28], large frontal sinuses [10,12,28] and high arched palate [53].

Heart manifestations

Cardiac involvement usually occurs late in the course of the disease and is rarely sufficient to cause cardiovascular signs or symptoms.

More frequently ECG abnormalities are found, the most common being disturbance of the atrioventricular conduction [14]. His bundle electrocardiography demonstrated abnormalities throughout the entire conducting system [30].

Pulmonary manifestations

Lung function varies greatly, depending on the degree of involvement of the respiratory muscles. Alveolar hypoventilation [15] and a gross reduction in the maximum expiratory pressure [27] were found.

There is a high risk during anaesthesia [55,65]. Thiopentone in particular may give rise to a prolonged depression of respiration.

Involvement of the nervous system

Mental defects, intellectual deterioration, lack of drive and initiative and increased need of sleep, are often present in varying degree. These features, together with the progressive muscular weakness, give rise to a steady social decline of many patients [19,66].

Non-specific electroencephalographic abnormalities and ventricular enlargement were also described.

The association of dystrophia myotonica with decreased motor nerve conduction velocities, or with clinical signs of polyneuropathy, has been observed in a number of patients [8,11,44,46,50]. For some unknown reason most of these patients were men [35].

Laboratory findings

There may be moderate increase of the serum CPK activity and creatinuria. Spinal fluid protein may be elevated in some cases.

Muscle pathology

Muscle biopsy findings consist of a marked variation in fibre size, increase of multiple internal nuclei, formation of long chains of nuclei, ringed fibres and sarcoplasmic masses. In early stages of the disease preferential atrophy of type I fibres can be seen [24]. Large type II fibres and groups of moth-eaten (or lobulated) fibres are a common finding.

The muscle spindles may show large numbers of very small intrafusal fibres, due to longitudinal splitting [36,64].

Electron microscopy revealed alteration of the sarcoplasmic reticulum in the early stages [43] and myofibrillar disorganisation in the more advanced stages of the disease.

The sarcoplasmic masses contain mitochondria, numerous ribosomes and polysomes, and irregularly orientated small bundles of myofilaments. This is suggestive of the regenerative nature of sarcoplasmic masses [43].

Genetic aspects

The disease is inherited as an autosomal dominant trait. There is a marked variation in expressivity as to severity and age of onset. A family in which the affected members were all females has been described [49].

Many patients are not aware that they are suffering from the disease.

Although, in each successive generation, the disease appears to start at an earlier age and seems to be more severe, most authors agree that this phenomenon of progression with anticipation in pedigrees of dystrophia myotonica is not a reality.

The most useful method for early recognition of symptomless heterozygotes is clinical examination [51]. Other methods for early detection [10,51] are electromyography (myotonic discharges), slit-lamp examination (cataract) and the estimation of plasma insulin response to oral glucose load (hypersecretion). Low immunoglobulin G serum levels, presumably due to an isolated hypercatabolism of IgG [71], may be of relative value in the detection of heterozygotes for the gene for the disease.

The use of linkage analysis in prenatal (examination of amniotic fluid) or postnatal prediction (examination of saliva) may also facilitate early diagnosis [33,61]. The dystrophia myotonica gene, the Lutheran blood group, and the gene which determines the ability to secrete ABH blood group substance in saliva and body fluids (the secretor gene), are situated close together on the same chromosome [34,56].

Pathogenesis
It has been proposed that the muscle involvement in dystrophia myotonica is secondary to chronic lower motor neuron involvement and that the disease is – at least in part – a form of neuropathy, and not a myopathy [23]. Also, it was proposed that a decrease of inhibitory influence from the lower motor neuron to the muscle is manifested as myotonia. This chronic, partial defect of neuronal influence on muscle can be a functional abnormality.

Electrophysiological study of the extensor digitorum brevis muscle, suggested a primary defect of the motor innervation in dystrophia myotonica [40].

With a computer method for the analysis of evoked motor unit potentials, it was found that there is a disturbance of function in the motor axons and intramuscular nerve fibres in this disease [5].

Using the methylene-blue technique it was seen that the motor endplates were enlarged, there was prominent sprouting of the distal part of the terminal axons [17] and abnormal swellings of axons and myelin [41]. An increase in the terminal innervation ratio was found in some cases [16]. Peripheral nerve morphometry carried out in 4 patients showed no evidence of morphologic abnormality of the peripheral nerves [52]. Morphometric analysis of the nerve terminals demonstrated a decreased mean synaptic vesicle density and an increased mean mitochondrial content of the nerve terminals. No abnormalities in the post-synaptic regions or intramuscular nerves were observed. These findings were not considered as evidence of a neurogenic etiology [22].

No increased extrajunctional acetylcholine receptor sites — measured by a technique utilizing ^{125}I-labelled alpha-bungarotoxin — were seen in muscle biopsies from 9 patients [20].

Other investigators concluded that the muscles and the nerves were independently affected by the pleiotropic gene of the disease [44,45].

Highly purified sarcolemma from patients with myotonic dystrophy showed a normal amount of phospholipids, but these contained more unsaturated fatty acids than normal. In addition a high phospholipid:cholesterol ratio was found, reflecting a relative decrease in cholesterol [47].

The platelets in patients with dystrophia myotonia were unusually sensitive to adrenaline, aggregation being detectable with very low adrenaline concentrations (0.041 μmol/l). It was thought that this increased sensitivity to adrenaline might be related to a decrease in phosphorylation of the platelet membrane.

The pattern of aggregation was normal in response to adenosine diphosphate [9]. In dystrophia myotonica patients, 20–80 per cent of the erythrocytes were cup-shaped (stomatocytes). Moreover, it was found that the erythrocytes showed membrane defects [57]. Because these erythrocyte membrane changes can have no primary myopathic, neurogenic or vascular cause, it was suggested that the defect of the muscle membrane is only part of a more widespread metabolic alteration of membranes in this disease. This possibilith has also been raised by the finding of an increase in the serum gamma-glutamyl transpeptidase activity. This membrane-bound enzyme is associated with cell membranes of different tissues, particularly in cells where high rates of amino acid transport are observed [3].

Neonatal dystrophia myotonica

This manifestation of the disease has also been called congenital [21,31], early onset [70] and infantile [38] dystrophia myotonica, and myotonic dysembryoplasia 54].

The syndrome is present at birth and is characterized by severe, generalized hypotonia and muscular weakness, facial diplegia and difficulties in breathing [1], sucking and swallowing. The deep tendon reflexes can usually be obtained [72]. Other features are: thin ribs [6,26], bilateral talipes and other congenital physical defects [21,31,54,67,70]. Reduction in foetal movements and the frequent occurrence of hydramnios may represent prenatal manifestations of the disorder [2,31].

Prognosis is often unfavourable and many patients die in the neonatal period. When they survive, the motor development is delayed, distal muscular weakness becomes apparent, the speech is nasal and dysarthic, and there is a high incidence of mental retardation. Usually myotonia cannot be elicited before the age of 2 years [38] but electromyographic myotonia has been observed in a 9-month-old patient [67], and myotonia after closure of the eyes was seen in a 1-year-old patient [70].

All patients have a parent with dystrophia myotonica, which is always the mother, who is usually only mildly affected. There is strong clinical evidence that this form of the disease results from a maternal intrauterine factor affecting those individuals carrying the dystrophia myotonica gene [32]. While the affected mothers have pursed lips, the patients with neonatal dystrophia myotonica have a characteristic tented upper lip that remains constant throughout life [21].

In neonatal dystrophia myotonica a marked variation in fibre diameter and type II fibre predominance without type I fibre hypotrophy, was observed. In addition, there was a light sarcoplasmic halo at the periphery of most fibres, best seen in sections stained for the activity of oxidative enzymes [25].

Electron microscopy of the region of the halo showed sarcoplasm with some myofilaments, glycogen granules, occasional triads and an almost complete absence of mitochondria. Some electron microscopic features, such as dilated transverse tubules that were aligned longitudinally, poorly formed Z discs, central nuclei containing fine granular chromatin and many satellite cells, were considered to be consistent with a maturational arrest in the myotubular stage of development [60].

In infancy, type I fibre hypotrophy but no type II fibre predominance was seen [38]. Most fibres showed, at the periphery near the nucleus, an increase in acid phosphatase activity. Ultrastructural studies of this area revealed disoriented myofilaments and dense core tubules, presumably the site of the acid phosphatase activity.

References   1   Aicardi,J.,Conti,D.,Goutières,F.
Les formes néo-natales de la dystrophie myotonique de Steinert.
J.neurol.Sci.1974,22:149–164.

2   Aicardi,J.,Conti,D.,Goutières,F.
Aspects cliniques et génétiques des formes precoces de la dystrophie myotonique de Steinert.
J.Génét.hum.1975,23,Suppl.:146–157

3   Alevizos,B.,Spengos,M.,Vassilopoulos,D.,Stefanis,C.
γ-Glutamyl transpeptidase. Elevated activity in myotonic dystrophy.
J.neurol.Sci.1976,28:225–231

4   Babel,J.
Fréquence des complications rétiniennes dans la dystrophie myotonique.
J.Génét.hum.1976,23,Suppl.:167–171

5   Ballantyne,J.P.,Hansen,S.
Computer method for the analysis of evoked motor unit

potentials. 2. Duchenne, limb-girdle, facioscapulohumeral
and myotonic muscular dystrophies.
J.Neurol.Neurosurg.Psychiat.1975,38:417–428

6   Bell,D.B.,Smith,D.W.
Myotonic dystrophy in the neonate.
J.Pediat.1972,81:83–86

7   Bethlem,J.
Dystrophia myotonica (ziekte van Steinert).
Thesis,Amsterdam,1955

8   Bethlem,J.
Observations on dystrophia myotonica.
In:Recent Neurological Research.A.Biemond(ed.).
Amsterdam,Elsevier,1959,pp.1–10

9   Bousser,M.G.,Lecrubier,C.,Conard,J.,Samama,M.
Increased sensitivity of platelets to adrenaline in human
myotonic dystrophy.
Lancet 1975,II:307–309

10 Bundey,S.,Carter,C.O.,Soothill,J.F.
Early recognition of heterozygotes for the gene for dystrophia
myotonica.
J.Neurol.Neurosurg.Psychiat.1970,33:279–293

11 Caccia,M.R.,Negri,S.,Parvis,V.P.
Myotonic dystrophy with neural involvement.
J.neurol.Sci.1972,16:253–269

12 Caughey,J.E.
Bone changes in the skull in dystrophia myotonica.
J.Bone Jt Surg.1952,34B:343–351

13 Caughey,J.E.,Myrianthopoulos,N.C.
Dystrophia Myotonica and Related Disorders.
Springfield,Ill.,Thomas,1963

14 Church,S.C.
The heart in myotonia atrophica.
Arch.intern.Med.1967,119:176–181

15 Coccagna,G.,Mantovani,M.,Parchi,C.,Mironi,F.,Lugaresi,E.
Alveolar hypoventilation and hypersomnia in myotonic
dystrophy.
J.Neurol.Neurosurg.Psychiat.1975,38:977–984

16 Coërs,C.,Telerman-Toppet,N.,Gérard,J.-M.
Terminal innervation ratio in neuromuscular disease.

II. Disorders of lower motor neuron, peripheral nerve, and muscle.
Arch.Neurol.(Chic.)1973,29:215–222

17 Coërs,C.,Woolf,A.L.
The Innervation of Muscle. A biopsy study.
Springfield,Ill.,Thomas,1959

18 Cudworth,A.G.,Walker,B.A.
Carbohydrate metabolism in dystrophia myotonica.
J.med.Genet.1975,12:157–161

19 DeJong,J.G.Y.
Dystrophia myotonica, paramyotonia en myotonia congenita.
Thesis,Utrecht,1955

20 Drachman,D.B.,Fambrough,D.M.
Are muscle fibers denervated in myotonic dystrophy?
Arch.Neurol.(Chic.)1976,33:485–488

21 Dyken,P.R.,Harper,P.S.
Congenital dystrophia myotonica.
Neurology (Minneap.)1973,23:465–473

22 Engel,A.G.,Jerusalem,F.,Tsujihata,M.,Gomez,M.R.
The neuromuscular junction in myopathies. A quantitative ultrastructural study.
In:Recent Advances in Myology. Proceedings of the 3rd International Congress on Muscle Diseases,Newcastle upon Tyne,15–21September1974.Amsterdam,Excerpta Medica,1974,pp.132–143.(Int.Congr.Ser.360)

23 Engel,W.K.
Myotonia – a different point of view.
Calif.Med.1971,114:32–37

24 Engel,W.K.,Brooke,M.H.
Histochemistry of the myotonic disorders.
In:Progressive Muskeldystrophie,Myotonie,Myasthenie.
E.Kuhn(ed.).Berlin,Springer,1966,pp.203–222

25 Farkas,E.,Tomé,F.M.S.,Fardeau,M.,Arsénio-Nunes,M.L.,
Dreyfus,P.,Diebler,M.F.
Histochemical and ultrastructural study of muscle biopsies in 3 cases of dystrophia myotonica in the newborn child.
J.neurol.Sci.1974,21:273–288

26 Fried,K.,Pajewski,M.,Mundel,G.,Caspl,E.,Spira,R.
Thin ribs in neonatal myotonic dystrophy.
Clin.Genet.1975,2:417–420

27   Gillam,P.M.S.,Heaf,P.J.D.,Kaufman,L.,Lucas,B.G.B.
      Respiration in dystrophia myotonica.
      Thorax 1964,19:112–120
28   Gleeson,J.A.,Swann,J.C.,Hughes,D.T.D.,Lee,F.I.
      Dystrophia myotonica – a radiological survey.
      Brit.J.Radiol.1967,40:96–100
29   Gorden,P.,Griggs,R.C.,Nissley,S.P.,Roth,J.,Engel,W.K.
      Studies of plasma insulin in myotonic dystrophy.
      J.Clin.Endocr.1969,29:684–690
30   Griggs,R.C.,Davis,R.J.,Anderson,D.C.,Dove,J.T.
      Cardiac conduction in myotonic dystrophy.
      Amer.J.Med.1975,59:37–42
31   Harper,P.S.
      Congenital myotonic dystrophy in Britain. I. Clinical aspects.
      Arch.Dis.Childh.1975,50:505–513
32   Harper,P.S.
      Congenital myotonic dystrophy in Britain. II. Genetic basis.
      Arch.Dis.Childh.1975,50:514–521
33   Harper,P.,Bias,W.B.,Hutchinson,J.R.,McKusick,V.A.
      ABH secretor status of the fetus: a genetic marker
      identifiable by amniocentesis.
      J.med.Genet.1971,8:438–440
34   Harper,P.S.,Rivas,M.L.,Bias,W.B.,Hutchinson,J.R.,Dyken,P.R.
      McKusick,V.A.
      Genetic linkage confirmed between the locus for myotonic
      dystrophy and the ABH-secretion and Lutheran blood group
      loci.
      Amer.J.hum.Genet.1972,24:310–316
35   Hausmanowa-Petrusewicz,I.,Jedrzejowka,H.,Rowinska,R.,
      Barkowska,J.
      Peroneal atrophies connected with myotonic dystrophies.
      Paper read at the IVèmes Journées internationales de
      pathologie neuro-musculaire,Marseille,16–18 September 1976
36   Heene,R.
      Histological and histochemical findings in muscle spindles
      in dystrophia myotonica.
      J.neurol.Sci.1973,18:369–372
37   Huff,T.A.,Horton,E.A.,Lebovitz,H.E.
      Abnormal insulin secretion in myotonic dystrophy.
      New Engl.J.Med.1967,277:837–841

38   Karpati,G.,Carpenter,S.,Watters,G.V.,Eisen,A.A.,Andermann,F.
Infantile myotonic dystrophy. Histochemical and electron
microscopic features in skeletal muscle.
Neurology(Minneap.)1973,23:1066–1077.

39   Klein,D.
La dystrophie myotonique (Steinert) et la myotonie
congénitale (Thomsen) en Suisse. Etude clinique, génétique
et démographique.
Genève,1957.Supplement to:J.Génét.hum.1958,vol.7

40   McComas,A.J.,Campbell,M.J.,Sica,R.E.P.
Electrophysiological study of dystrophia myotonica.
J.Neurol.Neurosurg.Psychiat.1971,34:132–139

41   MacDermot,V.
The histology of the neuromuscular junction in dystrophia
myotonica.
Brain 1961,84:75–84

42   Marshall,J.
Observations on endocrine function in dystrophia myotonica.
Brain 1959,82:221–231

43   Mussini,I.,DiMauro,S.,Angelini,C.
Early structural and biochemical changes in muscle in
dystrophia myotonica.
J.neurol.Sci.1970,10:585–604

44   Panayiotopoulos,C.P.,Scarpalezos,S.
Dystrophia myotonica. Peripheral nerve involvement and
pathogenetic implications.
J.neurol.Sci.1976,27:1–16

45   Panayiotopoulos,C.P.,Scarpalezos,S.
Muscular dystrophies and motoneuron diseases.
A comparative electrophysiologic study.
Neurology(Minneap.)1976,26:721–725

46   Paramesh,K.,Smith,B.H.,Kalyanaraman,K.
Early onset myotonic dystrophy in association with
polyneuropathy.
J.Neurol.Neurosurg.Psychiat.1975,38:1136–1139

47   Peter,J.B.,Fiehn,W.
Distinctive lipid abnormalities in sarcolemma from patients
with myotonic dystrophy.
Clin.Res.1972,20:192

48 Peterson,D.M.,BoundsJr,J.V.,Karnes,W.E.
Clinical observations on thyrotoxicosis coexisting with
myotonic dystrophy.
Proc.Mayo Clin.1976,51:176–179

49 Pierson,M.,Saborio,M.,Schmitt,J.,André,J.M.,André,M.,
Fortier,G.
Une famille de dystrophie myotonique de Steinert, forme
congénitale n'affectant que les filles.
J.Génét.hum.1975,23,Suppl.:180

50 Pilz,H.,Prill,A.,Volles,E.
Kombination von myotonischer Dystrophie mit 'idiopathischer'
Neuropathie. Mitteilung klinischer Befunde bei 10 Fällen mit
gleichzeitiger Proteinvermehrung im Liquor.
Z.Neurol.1974,206:253–265

51 Polgar,J.G.,Bradley,W.G.,Upton,A.R.M.,Anderson,J.,
Howat,J.M.L.,Petito,F.,Roberts,D.F.,Scopa,J.
The early detection of dystrophia myotonica.
Brain 1972,95:761–776

52 Pollock,M.,Dyck,P.J.
Peripheral nerve morphometry in myotonic dystrophy.
Arch.Neurol.(Chic.)1976,33:33–39

53 Pruzanski,W.
Congenital malformations in myotonic dystrophy.
Acta neurol.scand.1965,41:34–38

54 Pruzanski,W.
Variants of myotonic dystrophy in pre-adolescent life
(the syndrome of myotonic dysembryoplasia).
Brain 1966,89:563–568

55 Ravin,M.,Newmark,Z.,Saviello,G.
Myotonia dystrophica – an anaesthetic hazard. Two case
reports.
Analg.Curr.Res.1975,54:216–218

56 Renwick,J.H.,Bundey,S.E.,Ferguson-Smith,M.A.,Izatt,M.M.
Confirmation of linkage of the loci for myotonic dystrophy
and ABH secretion.
J.med.Genet.1971,8:407–416

57 Roses,A.D.,Butterfield,D.A.,Appel,S.H.,Chestnut,D.B.
Phenytoin and membrane fluidity in myotonic dystrophy.
Arch.Neurol.(Chic.)1975,32:535–538

58 Russell,D.,Sjaastad,O.
Biphasic response on oral glucose tolerance testing in myotonic dystrophy.
Acta neurol.scand.1976,53:226–228

59 Sagel,J.,Distiller,L.A.,Morley,J.E.,Isaacs,H.
Normal thyrotropin-releasing hormone response in myotonia dystrophica.
Arch.Neurol.(Chic.)1976,33:520

60 Sarnat,H.B.,Silbert,S.W.
Maturational arrest of fetal muscle in neonatal myotonic dystrophy. A pathologic study of four cases.
Arch.Neurol.(Chic.)1976,33:466–474

61 Schrott,H.G.,Omenn,G.S.
Myotonic dystrophy: opportunities for prenatal prediction.
Neurology(Minneap.)1975,25:789–791

62 Siegel,C.I.,Hendrix,T.R.,Harvey,J.C.
The swallowing disorder in myotonia dystrophica.
Gasteroenterology.1966,50:541–550

63 Stanescu,B.,Michiels,J.
Temporal aspects of electroretinography in patients with myotonic dystrophy.
Amer.J.Ophthal.1975,80:224–226

64 Swash,M.,Fox,K.P.
Abnormal intrafusal muscle fibers in myotonic dystrophy: a study using serial sections.
J.Neurol.Neurosurg.Psychiat.1975,38:91–99.

65 Telerman-Toppet,N.
Les accidents de narcose dans la dystrophie myotonique.
Acta neurol.belg.1970,70:551–560

66 Thomasen,E.
Myotonia. Thomsen's Disease (myotonia congenita), Paramyotonia, and Dystrophia Myotonica. A clinical and heredobiologic investigation.
Aarhus,Universitetsforlaget,1948

67 Vanier,T.M.
Dystrophia myotonica in childhood.
Brit.med.J.1960,11:1284–1288

68 Walsh,J.C.,Turtle,J.R.,Miller,S.,McLeod,J.G.
Abnormalities of insulin secretion in dystrophia myotonica.
Brain 1970,93:731–742

69   Walton,J.N.,Warrick,C.K.
         Osseous changes in myopathy.
         Brit.J.Radiol.1954,27:1–15
70   Watters,G.V.,Williams,T.W.
         Early onset myotonic dystrophy. Clinical and laboratory
         findings in five families and a review of the literature.
         Arch.Neurol.(Chic.)1967,17:137–152
71   Wochner,R.D.,Drews,G.,Strober,W.,Waldmann,T.A.
         Accelerated breakdown of immunoglobulin G (IgG) in
         myotonic dystrophy: a hereditary error of immunoglobin
         catabolism.
         J.clin.Invest.1966,45:321–329
72   Zellweger,H.,Ionasescu,V.
         Myotonic dystrophy of the neonate-inheritance and
         environment.
         J.Génét.hum.1975,23,Suppl.:182–185

Autosomal dominant type

This type is also called Thomsen's disease, after the Danish physician who himself suffered from the disorder. In 1876, he described it for the first time. The disease is inherited as an autosomal dominant trait, with high penetrance in both sexes.

The two main features consist of myotonia (page 141) and generalized hypertrophy of muscle.

Myotonia usually becomes manifest in infancy or childhood and in some cases is seen soon after birth in the orbicularis oculi muscles when the baby is sneezing and consequently closing the eyes. Action and percussion myotonia may be present in many muscles, but may vary in intensity from case to case or in the same patient. It is accentuated by exposure to cold, by rest, fatigue, menstruation, pregnancy and psychological factors. Sudden movements may cause generalized myotonia; climbing a stair may give rise to severe myotonia in the legs. In many patients myotonia is worse in puberty and decreases in advanced age.

The muscular hypertrophy is present in many patients and gives them an athletic appearance. It is especially seen in the gluteal, quadriceps and calf muscles, but the muscles of the neck, of the upper-arms and the deltoid muscles may also be markedly hypertrophic [7].

Muscle biopsy [3] shows slight, mainly non-specific changes. Complete absence of the type II B fibres has been described [2].

Myotonia can be relieved or abolished by administration of procainamide (1 mg, 3–4 times a day) or diphenylhydantoin (100 mg, 3–4 times a day). These drugs give less troublesome side-effects than quinine.

Autosomal recessive type

This type of myotonia congenita has been recognized by Becker [1] as a separate disease. In this disorder onset tends to be later than in Thomsen's disease, while myotonia is more severe. Myotonia is first present in the legs, it is only after some years that the upper extremities and finally the muscles of the face become affected.

In addition to the generalized muscular hypertrophy, there is weakness of both proximal and distal muscles [5].

Muscle histopathology and electron microscopy revealed no relevant abnormalities [4].

The differentiation of the two hereditary types of myotonia congenita is possible by biochemical assay of the muscle phosphatides. In the auto-somal recessive type, the fatty acid pattern of the muscle phosphatides is almost normal, while in the autosomal type there is a very marked abnormal pattern [6].

References   1   Becker,P.E.
Genetic approaches to the nosology of muscle disease:
myotonias and similar diseases.
Birth Def.,Orig.Art.Ser.1971,7:52–62

2   Dubowitz,V.,Brooke,M.H.
Muscle Biopsy. A modern approach.
Major Problems in Neurology;vol.2.London,Saunders,1973,
pp.229

3   Engel,W.K.,Brooke,M.H.
Histochemistry of the myotonic disorders.
In: Progressive Muskeldystrophie, Myotonie,Myasthenie.
E.Kuhn(ed.).Berlin,Springer,1966,pp.203–222

4   Fisher,E.R.,Danowski,T.S.,Ahmad,U.,Breslau,P.,Nolan,S.,
Stephan,T.
Electron microscopical study of a family with myotonia
congenita.
Arch.Path.1975,99:607–610

5   Harper,P.S.,Johnston,D.M.
Recessively inherited myotonia congenita.
J.med.Genet.1972,9:213–215

6   Kuhn,E.,Seiler,D.
Biochemische Besonderheiten und Unterschiede der
autosomal dominant und autosomal recessiv vererbten
Myotonia congenita.
Klin.Wschr.1970,48:1134–1136

7   Thomasen,E.
Myotonia.Thomsen's Disease (myotonia congenita),
Paramyotonia, and Dystrophia Myotonica. A clinical and
heredobiologic investigation.
Aarhus,Universitetsforlaget,1948

The name chondrodystrophic myotonia or osteo-chondro-muscular dystrophy was given to a syndrome consisting of dwarfism, skeletal deformities,
unusual facial abnormalities, blepharospasm and myotonia [1 and 9, 2 and
6,5,7,11]. It is also called Schwartz-Jampel syndrome [3,10] or Schwartz
syndrome [4,8].
The babies may be born with skeletal deformities but there are usually
no abnormalities at birth or soon after. The manifestations of the syndrome
become apparent in the first or second year of life.
All patients are dwarfs and they show slowly progressive bony deformities, including high-arched palates, coxa vara or valga — with marked irregularity along the articular surfaces and flattening of the femoral heads —
pigeon breast, reduction in the height of the vertebral bodies, scoliosis and
talipes equinovarus. In addition there is marked limitation of motion, due to
multiple joint contractures. There is a short neck, low set ears, a small re-
ceding chin and a very characteristic facial expression, with narrowed pal-
pebral apertures, a pursed mouth and blepharospasm with compensatory
over-activity of the frontal muscles, deep horizontal furrowing of the forehead and high arching of the eyebrows. The voice is high pitched, which was
found to be due to a marked hypoplasia of the larynx and abnormal shape
of the epiglottis [1]. Most patients are of normal intelligence.
Generalized muscular hypertrophy may be present, especially in boys
('infant Hercules' appearance). As a rule, muscle strength is within normal
limits, although muscular force is often very difficult to evaluate due to
the marked limitation of many joints.
In some patients, percussion myotonia can be a prominent feature and
in these cases it can be elicited in virtually all muscles [11] but it may be
absent in other patients [5].
Action myotonia may be present after closure of the eyes or after making
a fist. During electromyographic examination, myotonic discharges can be
easily elicited by movement of the needle after percussion of the muscle
or following voluntary contraction. In some patients electromyography
disclosed spontaneous activity ('neuromyotonia') as seen in continuous
muscle fibre activity [3,10].

The activity of serum creatine phosphokinase may be slightly elevated. Muscle biopsy may show no, or aspecific, abnormalities such as variation in fibre diameter and an increased number of sarcolemmal nuclei. There is a normal distribution of type I and type II fibres. In a patient with clinical signs of generalized muscular hypertrophy, there was a marked increase of the mean diameter of the muscle fibres [11]. Ultrastructural findings are also normal or non-specific.

Many of the patients so far described were brother and sister and were born to clinically normal parents. An autosomal recessive mode of inheritance is suggested by most authors.

References   1   Aberfeld,D.C.,Hinterbuchner,L.P.,Schneider,M.
Myotonia, dwarfism, diffuse bone disease and unusual ocular and facial abnormalities (a new syndrome).
Brain 1965,88:313–322

2   Aberfeld,D.C.,Namba,T.,Vye,M.V.,Grob,D.
Chondrodystrophic myotonia: report of two cases.
Myotonia, dwarfism, diffuse bone disease, and unusual ocular and facial abnormalities.
Arch.Neurol.(Chic.)1970,22:455–462

3   Cadilhac,J.,Baldet,P.,Greze,J.,Duday,H.
E.M.G. studies of two family cases of the Schwartz and Jampel syndrome. (Osteo-chondro-muscular dystrophy with myotonia).
Electromyogr.clin.Neurophysiol.1975,15:5–12

4   Cordeiro-Ferreira,N.,GomesdaCosta,M.G.,AmparoMarques,D.
Syndrôme de Schwartz.
Bordeaux Méd.1973,6:1777–1786

5   Huttenlocher,P.R.,Landwirth,J.,Hanson,V.,Gallagher,B.B.,Bensch,K.
Osteo-chondro-muscular dystrophy. A disorder manifested by multiple skeletal deformities, myotonia, and dystrophic changes in muscle.
Pediatrics 1969,44:945–958

6   Mereu,T.R.,Porter,I.H.,Hug,G.
Myotonia, shortness of stature, and hip dysplasia.

Schwartz-Jampel syndrome.
Amer.J.Dis.Child.1969,117:470–478

7 Pearson,C.M.,Kar,N.C.,Peter,J.B.,Munsat,T.L.,Fowler,W.M.,
Coleman,R.F.
Myotonic dystrophy. Its variable clinical, histochemical and
biochemical expressions.
In:Progress in Neurogenetics.A.Barbeau,J.R.Brunette(eds.).
Amsterdam,Excerpta Medica,1969,pp.199–218

8 Saadat,M.,Mokfi,H.,Vakil,H.,Ziai,M.
Schwartz syndrome: myotonia with blepharophimosis and
limitation of joints.
J.Pediat.1972,81:348–350

9 Schwartz,O.,Jampel,R.S.
Congenital blepharophimosis associated with a unique
generalized myopathy.
Arch.Ophthal.1962,68:82–87

10 Taylor,R.G.,Layzer,R.B.,Davis,H.S.,FowlerJr,W.M.
Continuous muscle fiber activity in the Schwartz-Jampel
syndrome.
Electroenceph.clin.Neurophysiol.1972,33:497–509

11 VanHuffelen,A.C.,Gabreëls,F.J.M.,VanLuypen-V.d.Horst,J.S.,
Slooff,J.L.,Stadhouders,A.M.,Korten,J.J.
Chondrodystrophic myotonia. A report of two unrelated
Dutch patients.
Neuropädiatrie 1974,1:71–90

In the periodic paralyses, the patients have paroxysmal attacks of transient flaccid paralysis of the extremities and, to a lesser extent, of the other musculature.

Recovery from the attacks is complete, but some patients may gradually develop persistent muscular weakness.

The following periodic paralyses can be recognized:

Autosomal dominantly inherited types
1. Hypokalaemic periodic paralysis (page 172);
2. Hyperkalaemic periodic paralysis or paramyotonia congenita (Eulenburg) or adynamia episodica hereditaria (Gamstorp) (page 175);
3. Normokalaemic periodic paralysis (page 180).

Sporadic, non-familial types (page 183)
1. Hypokalaemic periodic paralysis;
2. Hyperkalaemic periodic paralysis.

Differential diagnosis is very difficult because the three hereditary types of periodic paralysis have many features in common. Clinical characteristics of the attacks, such as age of onset, frequency, severity and duration, time of the day when paralysis occurs, precipitation by rest after exertion and the possibility to 'walk off' an incipient attack, may be more or less similar in all three forms. The features of a particular type of periodic paralysis can be fairly constant within the same family, but may vary markedly in different families.

Electrophysiological examination of single muscle fibres in hyperkalaemic and normokalaemic periodic paralysis have shown similar results: abnormally low resting membrane potentials and reduced membrane time constants [4].

Light and electron microscopy may show identical alterations in the three types, viz. vacuoles, tubular aggregates (page 170), dilatation of the longitudinal elements of the sarcoplasmic reticulum and increased muscle glycogen [2].

In all three forms treatment with the diuretic agent acetazolamide, a carbonic anhydrase inhibitor, has been effective.

However, the estimation of the plasma potassium concentration in blood draining a limb that is paralysed during a spontaneous, severe attack, may lead to a correct diagnosis.

According to Becker [1] there is a separate disease, viz. paralysis periodica paramyotonica, and he believes that this disease, adynamia episodica hereditaria and paramyotonia congenita are different, genetically independent disorders (page 142).

The fundamental defect in the familial periodic paralyses is not clear. The role of potassium in the pathogenesis of this group of diseases remains obscure.

Of differential diagnostic importance for the sporadic cases is the presence of periodic attacks of severe quadriparesis in patients who showed a myopathy with abnormal mitochondria and marked craving for salt (page 131). Attacks of muscular weakness may also be present in patients with lipid storage disease (page 215).

Periodic episodes of generalized muscle pain and weakness were present in a patient suffering from a disease characterized by intermittent muscle membrane disorder, resulting in muscle destruction [3]. During the attacks there was marked excretion of potassium, phosphorus, nitrogen and creatine, with normal plasma potassium level.

References   1   Becker,P.E.
Paramyotonia congenita (Eulenburg).
Stuttgart,Thieme,1970.(Fortschritte der allgemeinen und
klinischen Humangenetik;Bd.III)

2   Bradley,W.G.
Ultrastructural changes in adynamia episodica hereditaria and
normokalaemic familial periodic paralysis.
Brain 1969,92:379–390

3   Jacox,R.F.,Waterhouse,C.,Tobin,R.
Periodic disease associated with muscle destruction.
Amer.J.Med.1973,55:105–110

4   McComas,A.J.,Mrozek,K.,Bradley,W.G.
The nature of the electrophysiological disorder in adynamia
episodica.
J.Neurol.Neurosurg.Psychiat.1968,31:448–452

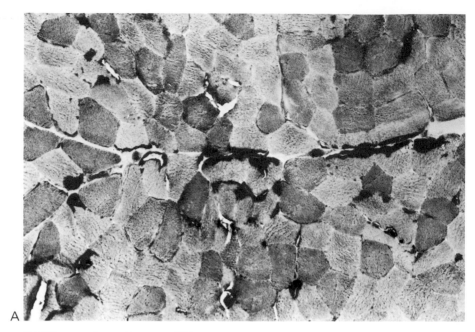

NADH-tetrazolium reductase, × 135

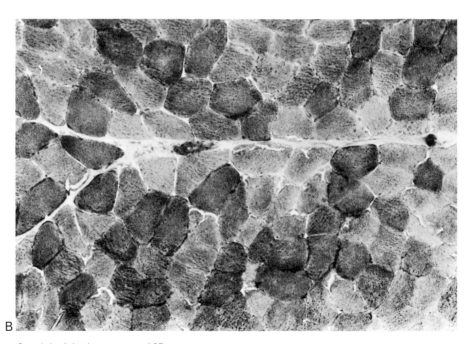

Succinic dehydrogenase, × 135

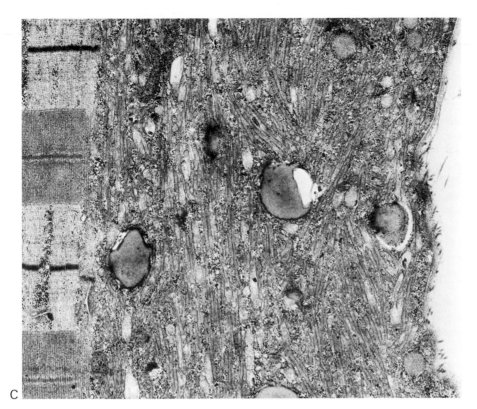

C

×17,554; figure kindly supplied by Dr.K.P. Dingemans

Tubular aggregates are most abundant in the muscle biopsies of patients suffering from one of the familial periodic paralyses (page 167), but they have been described in many other neuromuscular diseases and in normal individuals who had taken large amounts of various drugs over a long period of time.

They are only seen in the type II fibres and are usually present in the sub-sarcolemmal regions. They stain bright red with the modified Gomori trichrome method and show a high activity of all the oxidative enzymes, except succinic dehydrogenase and menadione-linked alpha-glycero-phosphate dehydrogenase.

Section A is stained for the activity of NADH-tetrazolium reductase. The tubular aggregates are present in the (lighter stained) type II fibres and show a strong reaction.

No reaction is seen in a serial section B, stained for the activity of succinic dehydrogenase.

Electron microscopy indicates that the aggregates are composed of closely packed clusters of long tubules (C).

Some authors consider the tubules as proliferated components of the sarcoplasmic reticulum, while others think they are of mitochondrial origin.

Familial hypokalaemic periodic paralysis is an autosomal dominantly inherited disease, in which males are affected more frequently than females. It is by far the most common of the periodic paralyses.

The onset of the first attacks is usually between 15 and 25 years of age. The attack occurs at night, and the patient awakens with a flaccid paralysis of the muscles of the trunk and extremities. During an attack the patient is as a rule able to talk, swallow, chew food and move the eyes, while respiration is seldom affected. Death in an attack may occur but is very rare.

In mild attacks the muscles are partially paralysed, weakness is less widespread and tends to be most severe in the proximal muscles of the legs. The reflexes are diminished or absent.

Excessive perspiration and thirst before and during an attack are prominent symptoms. The duration and frequency of the attacks differ widely, lasting from one hour to one week or more, and varying from several times a week to only once a year.

Usually the number of attacks increases till the fourth decade and then gradually decreases. In advanced age many patients may not experience any attacks at all.

Attacks may be precipitated by prolonged rest after strenuous exercise, excessive carbohydrate ingestion, cold and emotional stress. They can be provoked by the administration of sodium chloride, adrenalin, glucose and insulin.

An incipient attack may be relieved, postponed or prevented by continuing to engage in mild exercise and hence 'walking off' the muscular weakness.

The paralysed muscles are completely inexcitable to electrical stimulation. Although no hyperpolarization is present, action potential propagation fails. It has been shown [5] that the failure in excitation–contraction coupling resides in the surface membranous components of the muscle fibre, i.e. the surface membrane, the t-system and the sarcoplasmic reticulum.

During an attack prolonged indirect stimulation of a paralysed muscle results in complete recovery of evoked potential amplitude and clinical strength [1]. This is confined to the stimulated muscle only, while cessation of stimulation is immediately followed by the return of paralysis. This compares with the clinical finding where muscle activity may ward off an impending attack.

During an attack there is a low plasma potassium level (2–3.5 mEq/l) and a diminished urinary excretion of potassium. Although there is no loss of potassium from the body, there is a shift of potassium from the extracellular to the intracellular compartment. Weakness may become apparent even when the plasma potassium level is only slightly below normal, and which in normal subjects would produce no weakness.

Electrocardiography during an attack shows features of potassium depletion as in normal subjects, i.e. lowering of T waves and prolongation of PR, QRS and QT intervals.

Between the attacks many patients show no neurological abnormalities but some may have myotonic lid lag [8,9]. Persistent muscular weakness and atrophy – considered to be of myopathic origin – may develop, even in young patients [2,6]. This weakness is mainly proximal, the legs being more involved than the arms.

Muscle biopsy during an episode of weakness shows small vacuoles in the fibres, which may contain PAS-positive material. Light microscopy may reveal tubular aggregates in type II fibres. Both during and between attacks, ultrastructural studies [3,4,7,8] show dilatation of the terminal cisternae of the longitudinal component of the sarcoplasmic reticulum and tubular aggregates (page 170).

Attacks can be treated successfully by administration of potassium (5–10 g KCl) but the results of prophylactic potassium therapy are unsatisfactory. Acetazolamide (250–750 mg/day) can prevent attacks and even produce improvement of persistent weakness [6]. The mechanism of the effect of this kaliuretic drug is not understood. It produces metabolic acidosis and this may be responsible for the beneficial action [6,10,11].

References   1   Campa,J.F.,Sanders,D.B.
Familial hypokalemic periodic paralysis. Local recovery after nerve stimulation.
Arch.Neurol.(Chic.)1974,31:110–115

2 Dyken,M.,Zeman,W.,Rusche,T.
Hypokalemic periodic paralysis. Children with permanent myopathic weakness.
Neurology(Minneap.)1969,19:691–699

3 Engel,A.G.
Electron microscopic observations in primary hypokalemic and thyrotoxic periodic paralysis.
Proc.Mayo Clin.1966,41:797–808

4 Engel,A.G.
Evolution and content of vacuoles in primary hypokalemic periodic paralysis.
Proc.Mayo Clin.1970,45:774–814

5 Engel,A.G.,Lambert,E.H.
Calcium activation of electrically inexcitable muscle fibers in primary hypokalemic periodic paralysis.
Neurology(Minneap.)1969,19:851–858

6 Griggs,R.C.,Engel,W.K.,Resnick,J.S.
Acetazolamide treatment of hypokalemic periodic paralysis. Prevention of attacks and improvement of persistent weakness.
Ann.intern.Med.1970,73:39–48

7 HowesJr,E.L.,Price,H.M.,Pearson,C.M.,Blumberg,J.M.
Hypokalemic periodic paralysis. Electromicroscopic changes in the sarcoplasm.
Neurology(Minneap.)1966,16:242–256

8 Odor,D.L.,Patel,A.N.,Pearce,L.A.
Familial hypokalemic periodic paralysis with permanent myopathy. A clinical and ultrastructural study.
J.Neuropath.exp.Neurol.1967,26:98–114

9 Resnick,J.S.,Engel,W.K.
Myotonic lid lag in hypokalaemic periodic paralysis.
J.Neurol.Neurosurg.Psychiat.1967,30:47–51

10 Viskoper,R.J.,Licht,A.,Fidel,J.,Chaco,J.
Acetazolamide treatment in hypokalemic periodic paralysis: a metabolic and electromyographic study.
Amer.J.med.Sci.1973,266:119–123

11 Vroom,F.Q.,Jarrell,M.A.,Maren,T.H.
Acetazolamide treatment of hypokalemic periodic paralysis.
Arch.Neurol.(Chic.)1975,32:385–392

Familial hyperkalaemic periodic paralysis is an autosomal dominantly inherited disease, in which both sexes are equally affected. It is also known
as paramyotonia congenita (Eulenburg) depending on the predominant
symptoms.

In 1956, the disease was called adynamia episodica hereditaria by the
Swedish investigator Ingrid Gamstorp [6]. Members from branches of
the same pedigrees had already been reported on by other Scandinavian
authors: Kulneff (1902) and Helweg-Larsen, Haage and Sagild (1955).
In 1958 Drager, Hammill and Shy [4] suggested that paramyotonia congenita (Eulenburg) and adynamia episodica hereditaria were identical
diseases, a view that at present is accepted by most authors [8].

Additional synonyms are: familial hyperkalaemic paralysis with myotonia
and familial myotonic periodic paralysis.

Onset is usually in the first two decades of life.

The name **paramyotonia congenita** is used when myotonia is a prominent feature, and when this phenomenon together with attacks of muscular
weakness are precipitated by exposure to cold. The muscles of the face and
hands are then especially affected. The face becomes 'rigid', the eyelids
are partially closed, the intrinsic muscles of the hands become stiff and
the fingers are flexed and abducted. This is followed by flaccid paralysis
of the intrinsic muscles. These features resolve when the patient is exposed
to a warm environment.

Myotonia of the face and hands, brought on by exposure to cold, increases
further during repetitive contractions of the involved muscles (myotonia
paradoxa). According to Magee [10,11], the primary clinical abnormality
in paramyotonia congenita is paradoxical myotonia, followed by localized
weakness. With sufficient exercise myotonia can always be produced,
even at high temperatures (37.0 °C). This phenomenon is only 'catalyzed'
by exposure to cold, and in these circumstances the amount of exertion,
necessary to produce symptoms, is markedly decreased.

At any temperature percussion myotonia of the tongue and myotonic lid
lag can be present, and, less frequently, delayed opening of the vigorously
closed eyes or fist.

The name **adynamia episodica hereditaria** [6] is used when attacks of generalized paralysis, especially involving the trunk and extremities, are predominating the clinical picture.

As a rule the attacks occur during the day. The duration of the attack is usually short (one hour) but may vary widely, from minutes to months, and the frequency ranges from once a day to once a year. During an attack there is weakness or complete flaccid paralysis of the muscles of the extremities; the proximal muscles of the lower limbs are preferentially involved. Weakness of bulbar and respiratory muscles is far less frequent.

The deep tendon reflexes are decreased or absent during an attack. In addition there may be a positive Chvostek sign.

Attacks are precipitated by rest after strenuous exercise, cold, fasting, emotional stress and oral ingestion of potassium (approximately 5 g KCl). Many patients can prevent an incipient attack by taking bread or sugar ('eat it off') and by gentle exercise ('walk it off').

During an attack there is a shift of potassium from the muscle into the plasma and consequently the plasma potassium level is raised (5–7 mEq/l). This is associated with increased urinary potassium output. The rise of plasma potassium concentration is insufficient to produce muscular weakness in normal persons. In some attacks the potassium level may remain normal or even be below normal [12]. However, it has been found that a raised plasma potassium concentration may be found only in the blood draining paralysed muscles [1].

In patients with hyperkalaemic periodic paralysis, ribosomes, isolated from the muscle during KCl-induced attacks, showed definite increase of protein synthesis in a group of rather heavy muscle polyribosomes [7].

Between attacks, signs of myotonia may be found, but the severity of this phenomenon may vary in different families or in different members of the same family [8]. In one family, signs of myotonia were not evident until after treatment with diuretics [3]. Electromyography between attacks may show high frequency discharges and fibrillation potentials [8].

There is no apparent correlation between the severity of myotonia and the paralytic attacks. In some patients persistent, mainly proximal, muscular weakness and atrophy may be present, especially after the fourth decade. Muscle biopsy may show slight non-specific features, but a marked variation in fibre diameter [13] and the presence of target fibres [5] have been described.

Vacuoles and subsarcolemmal blebs with excess of glycogen can be present, especially when the biopsy has been taken during an attack. Histochemical examination and electron microscopy may show tubular aggregates (page 170).

Between attacks, ultrastructural studies show dilatation of the longitudinal elements of the sarcoplasmic reticulum and an increase of glycogen in the region of the I bands [2].

Muscular weakness during an attack can be terminated by intramuscular injection of calcium gluconate [14] or of agents that produce intracellular potassium shift, such as adrenalin or norepinephrine [3]. Attacks can be prevented by agents that promote urinary diuresis of potassium (and sodium). These include acetazolamide, dichlorphenamide, chlorothiazide and hydrochlorothiazide [3,8,9]. When taken at the beginning of an attack, 2–4 inhalations of salbutamol (200–400 µg) results in prompt alleviation of the hyperkalaemia and muscular weakness [15]. This method has the advantage that the patient does not have to take medicine daily. Moreover, the long-term administration of acetazolamide may give rise to kidney stones.

References   **1**   Bradley,W.G.
                           Adynamia episodica hereditaria. Clinical, pathological and
                           electrophysiological studies in an affected family.
                           Brain 1969,92:345–378
                  2   Bradley,W.G.
                           Ultrastructural changes in adynamia episodica hereditaria
                           and normokalaemic familial periodic paralysis.
                           Brain 1969,92:379–390
                  3   Carson,M.J.,Pearson,C.M.

Familial hyperkalemic periodic paralysis with myotonic features.
J.Pediat.1964,64:853–865

4   Drager,G.A.,Hammill,J.F.,Shy,G.M.
Paramyotonia congenita.
Arch.Neurol.Psychiat(Chic.)1958,80:1–9

5   Engel,W.K.
The essentiality of histo- and cytochemical studies of skeletal muscle in the investigation of neuromuscular disease.
Neurology(Minneap.)1962,12:778–794

6   Gamstorp,I.
Adynamia episodica hereditaria.
Lund,1956.Suppl.to Acta paediat.

7   Ionasescu,V.,Zellweger,H.,Schochet Jr,S.S.,Conway,T.W.
Biochemical abnormalities of muscle ribosomes during attacks of hyperkalemic periodic paralysis.
J.neurol.Sci.1973,19:389–398

8   Layzer,R.B.,Lovelace,R.E.,Rowland,L.P.
Hyperkalemic periodic paralysis.
Arch.Neurol.(Chic.)1967,16:455–472

9   McArdle,B.
Adynamia episodica hereditaria and its treatment.
Brain 1962,85:121–148

10   Magee,K.R.
A study of paramyotonia congenita.
Arch.Neurol.(Chic.)1963,8:461–470

11   Magee,K.R.
Paramyotonia congenita. Association with cutaneous cold sensitivity and description of peculiar sustained postures after muscle contraction.
Arch.Neurol.(Chic.)1966,14:590–594

12   Pearson,C.M.
The periodic paralysis: differential features and pathological observations in permanent myopathic weakness.
Brain 1964,87:341–354

13   Thrush,D.C.,Morris,C.J.,Salmon,M.V.
Paramyotonia congenita: a clinical, histochemical and pathological study.
Brain 1972,95:537–552

14 Van'tHoff,W.
Familial myotonic periodic paralysis.
Quart.J.Med.1962,31 : 385–402

15 Wang,P.,Clausen,T.
Treatment of attacks in hyperkalaemic familial periodic
paralysis by inhalation of salbutamol.
Lancet 1976,I :221–223

In 1951 Tyler, Stephens, Gunn and Perkoff [6] gave the first description of a pedigree in which 33 members in seven generations were suffering from periodic paralysis. There was no correlation between the attacks and the plasma potassium concentration.

The pattern of inheritance was that of an autosomal dominant trait with complete penetrance.

Onset of the initial attack in this pedigree was in the first year of life, and often in the first months of life. There was a tendency for the frequency of the episodes of weakness or flaccid paralysis to increase during child-hood and adolescense, and to decrease with advancing age. The duration of the attacks varied from a few minutes to several days, and they generally occurred in the early morning. They were most consistently produced by strenuous exercise followed by complete rest. Paralysis did not occur when the patient tried to 'walk off' an incipient attack by continuing muscular activity. A heavy meal or the ingestion of a large amount of carbohydrate, especially if taken before bedtime, sometimes produced an attack on the following morning. No patient reported attacks, precipitated by high carbohydrate intake, within two hours of ingestion. Between attacks all patients showed a slight but definite weakness of the extensors of the arms and legs, in addition to an increased muscle bulk, especially of the calf muscles and the extensors of the arms.

Biopsy of the enlarged gastrocnemius muscles in three patients showed vacuoles in the centre of some fibres, sometimes containing granules that stained red with the Best's carmine staining method.

During the episodes of mild or severe paralysis no significant change in the plasma potassium, sodium or magnesium levels was found.

Ten years later, Poskanzer and Kerr [5] reported another large family in which 22 members suffered from an autosomal dominantly inherited type of periodic paralysis in which the plasma potassium concentration was normal during the attacks. The onset of symptoms was between 2 and 10 years of age. During an attack — which started mainly at night — the patients were quadriplegic and often had facial weakness, difficulty in chewing food and a weak cough. In many patients the paralysis was asymmetrical, and often the most frequently used muscles were the most severely affected.

The duration of the paralysis varied from 2 days to 3 weeks. Physical examination revealed no abnormalities between the attacks.

In these patients an attack could be precipitated by rest after strenuous exertion or by sleeping late in the morning ('sunday morning paralysis'). The patients were able to prevent paralysis by walking or gentle exercise. Ingestion of a heavy meal or high carbohydrate intake could neither produce nor ward off an attack.

Administration of potassium chloride could provoke paralysis or exacerbate a mild attack. Because many members had a history of consistent high salt intake, the effect of administration of sodium chloride was examined and proved to be very useful in treating attacks of paralysis. Attacks were also prevented by daily administration of a combination of 0.1 mg of 9-alpha-fluorohydrocortisone (which causes retention of sodium and chloride) and 250 mg of the diuretic agent acetazolamide (a carbonic anhydrase inhibitor that promotes the excretion of potassium).

In two patients, originally described by Poskanzer and Kerr, later electron-microscopic studies of the muscle tissue, taken between attacks, showed dilatation of the longitudinal elements of the sarcoplasmic reticulum, increased glycogen and tubular aggregates (page 170; [2]). Similar ultra-structural changes have been found in hypo- and hyperkalaemic periodic paralysis.

Examination between attacks revealed no clinical findings in 2 patients [4] in whom the onset was in the second decade of life. There was a consistent elevation of the activity of serum creatine phosphokinase in these patients. Light microscopy of the type II fibres of one of these cases showed tubular aggregates.

A reappraisal of patients with normokalaemic periodic paralysis has been suggested by Bradley [1]. He found, in adynamia episodica hereditaria, that while the plasma potassium concentration was raised in venous blood draining the paralysed muscles, it was sometimes normal when estimated in antecubital venous blood during paralysis restricted to the muscles of the legs. Moreover, there is a striking similarity between normokalaemic periodic paralysis and adynamia episodica hereditaria [1] and between normokalaemic and hypokalaemic periodic paralysis [3].

References   1   Bradley,W.G.
Adynamia episodica hereditaria. Clinical, pathological and electrophysiological studies in an affected family.
Brain 1969,92:345–378

2   Bradley,W.G.
Ultrastructural changes in adynamia episodica hereditaria and normokalaemic familial periodic paralysis.
Brain 1969,92:379–390

3   Kusakabe,T.,Shiotu,H.,Nishikawa,M.
Metabolic studies on a case of paroxysmal myotonia with periodic paralysis.
Metabolism 1974,23:215–223

4   Meyers,K.R.,Gilden,D.H.,Rinaldi,C.F.,Hansen,J.L.
Periodic muscle weakness, normokalaemia, and tubular aggregates.
Neurology(Minneap.)1972,22:269–279·

5   Poskanzer,D.C.,Kerr,D.N.S.
A third type of periodic paralysis, with normokalemia and favourable response to sodium chloride.
Amer.J.Med.1961,31:328–342

6   Tyler,F.H.,Stephens,F.E.,Gunn,F.D.,Perkoff,G.T.
Studies in disorders of muscle VII. Clinical manifestations and inheritance of a type of periodic paralysis without hypopotassemia.
J.clin.Invest.1951,30:492–502

Sporadic cases of hypokalaemic periodic paralysis have been reported by many authors. Such cases may be associated with thyrotoxicosis. This association is especially seen in Oriental patients, in whom the incidence of periodic paralysis in hyperthyroidism was found to be up to 8 per cent [11]. Males are more frequently involved then females [8,11] while the age at onset of the paralytic attacks is in the second or third decade. The onset of the attacks coincided with or followed the onset of hyper-thyroidism in most patients. Successful treatment of the hyperthyroidism nearly always led to cessation of the attacks.

There seems to be a latent defect in these patients, which becomes evident only in the presence of excessive thyroid hormone. In some cases this latent defect may be hereditary [7]. The mechanism by which hyperthyroidism predisposes the patients to periodic paralysis is not known. Hyperactivity of the sympathetic nervous system appeared not to be an essential feature of this mechanism [10]. During an attack there is a decrease in calcium uptake and ATPase activity of the sarcoplasmic reticulum [1,12]. The clinical features of these hypokalaemic paralytic attacks are identical to those of the familial disease, while the light and electron microscopic findings in the muscle are also similar [2,12].

Episodes of periodic paralysis may also develop in patients who are taking thyroid hormone in order to lose weight [5].

Attacks of muscle weakness may be one of the most common presenting features in primary aldosteronism. These patients, however, have hyperten-sion, headache, polydipsia, nocturnal polyuria and alkalosis. The excessive aldosterone secretion results in hypokalaemia due to the marked renal loss of potassium.

Muscular weakness in severe hypokalaemia due to gastro-intestinal [3] and urinary potassium loss [14], can readily be differentiated from periodic paralysis. The use of laxatives, diuretics, licorice [13] and carbenoxolone sodium [9] have to be considered in these patients. A remarkable finding was the patient with hypokalaemic periodic paralysis and myotonia, who came from a family where the other members suffered from dystrophia myotonica [6].

Sporadic cases of hyperkalaemic periodic paralysis are very rare. Attacks of flaccid paralysis, predominantly involving the lower extremities, can occur in hyperkalaemia present in patients suffering from Addison's disease [4].

References   1   Au,K.-S.,Yeung,R.T.T.
Thyrotoxic periodic paralysis. Periodic variation in the
muscle calcium pump activity.
Arch.Neurol.(Chic.)1972,26:543–546

2   Bergman,R.A.,Afifi,A.K.,Dunkle,L.M.,Johns,R.J.
Muscle pathology in hypokalemic periodic paralysis with
hyperthyroidism. II. A light and electron microscopic study.
Johns Hopk.med.J.1970,126:100–118

3   Coërs,C.,Telerman-Toppet,N.,Cremer,M.
Acute quadriparesis with muscle spasms related to
disturbances in steatorrhea. Clinical and biochemical data.
Amer.J.Med.1972,52:849–856

4   Duc,M.,Duc,M.L.,Mauuary,G.
Paralysies intermittentes pas hyperkalémie révélatrices
d'une maladie d'Addison.
Ann.méd.Nancy.1970,9:387–390

5   Layzer,R.B.,Goldfield,E.
Periodic paralysis caused by abuse of thyroid hormone.
Neurology(Minneap.)1974,24:949–952

6   Leyburn,P.,Walton,J.N.
The effect of changes in serum potassium upon myotonia.
J.Neurol.Neurosurg.Psychiat.1960,23:119–126

7   McFadzean,A.J.S.,Yeung,R.
Familial occurrence of thyrotoxic periodic paralysis.
Brit.med.J.1969,1:760

8   Okinaka,S.,Shizume,K.,Iino,S.,Watanabe,A.,Irie,M.,
Noguchi,A.,Kuma,S.,Kuma,K.,Ito,T.
The association of periodic paralysis and hyperthyroidism in
Japan.
J.clin.Endocr.1957,17:1454–1459

9   Rankin,J.,Scott,M.E.
Hypokalaemic paralysis due to carbenoxolone.
Ulster med.J.1973,42:84–86

10   Resnick,J.S.,Dorman,J.D.,Engel,W.K.
     Thyrotoxic periodic paralysis.
     Amer.J.Med.1969,47:831—836

11   Satoyoshi,E.,Murakami,K.,Kowa,H.,Kinoshita,M.,Nishiyama,Y.
     Periodic paralysis in hyperthyroidism.
     Neurology(Minneap.)1963,13:746—752

12   Takagi,A.,Schotland,D.L.,DiMauro,S.,Rowland,L.P.
     Thyrotoxic periodic paralysis.
     Neurology(Minneap.)1973,23:1008—1016

13   Tourtelotte,C.R.,Hirst,A.E.
     Hypokalaemia, muscle weakness, and myoglobinuria due to
     licorice ingestion.
     Calif.Med.1970,113:51—53

14   VanHorn,G.,Drori,J.B.,Schwartz,F.D.
     Hypokalemic myopathy and elevation of serum enzymes.
     Arch.Neurol.(Chic.)1970,22:335—341

Glycogen storage diseases

Type	Enzyme deficiency	Other nomenclature	Clinical involvement of muscle
I	glucose-6-phosphatase	von Gierke's disease	no
II	acid maltase (acid alpha-1,4-gluco-sidase)	Pompe's disease	yes
III	amylo-1,6-glucosidase (debranching enzyme)	Cori's disease Forbes' disease Limit dextrinosis	yes
IV	amylo-1,4 → 1,6-transglucosidase (α-1,4-glucan 6-glycosyl transferase or branching enzyme)	Andersen's disease Amylopectinosis	yes
V	muscle phosphorylase	McArdle's disease	yes
VI	liver phosphorylase	Hers' disease	no
VII	phosphofructokinase	Tarui's disease	yes
VIII	liver phosphorylase b kinase	–	possible

The glycogen storage diseases or glycogenoses are a group of diseases in which there is an inborn error of glycogen metabolism. The numerical classification by Cori (1957) has been used for many years, although the name of the author who first described the disorder has often been attached to the disease. The best appellation of the different types of glycogen storage diseases seems to be that in which the name of the underlying enzyme deficiency is used (table).

At present the following enzymatic defects are thought to cause glycogen storage in one or several organs:

Glucose-6-phosphatase deficiency (type I; von Gierke's disease) There is no involvement of the muscles and no neurological symptoms are present. In this disease bodily growth is retarded and the liver is grossly enlarged.

Acid maltase deficiency (type II; Pompe's disease; acid alpha-1,4-glucosidase deficiency) (page 191)

Debranching enzyme deficiency (type III; Cori's disease; Forbes' disease; amylo-1,6-glucosidase deficiency; limit dextrinosis) (page 196)

Branching enzyme deficiency (type IV; Andersen's disease; amylo-1,4 → 1,6-transglucosidase deficiency; alpha-1,4-glucan 6-glycosyl transferase deficiency; amylopectinosis) (page 199)

Muscle phosphorylase deficiency (type V; McArdle's disease) (page 202)

Liver phosphorylase deficiency (type VI; Hers' disease) There is hepatomegaly without involvement of the skeletal muscles.

Phosphofructokinase deficiency (type VII; Tarui's disease) (page 206)

Liver phosphorylase b kinase deficiency (type VIII)
In the first years of life there is retarded growth and developmental delay. Hepatomegaly of varying degree and fasting hypoglycaemia are found. Mild muscular weakness and elevation of the activity of serum creatine phosphokinase may occur [1]. After puberty, all features tend to remit and most adult patients have no symptoms. This type of glycogen storage disease is X-linked and the locus involved is subject to X inactivation [4].

In addition, other glycogen storage diseases have been described in which the inborn error in less definite. Insufficiency of *phosphoglucomutase* and possible other glycolytic enzymes [10] was suggested, but not proved, in a 4-year-old boy with generalized mild muscular weakness. He showed uncommonly bulky and firm gastrocnemius muscles with contractures giving rise to plantar-flexion deformities of the feet. There was only a very slight rise of blood lactate after ischaemic exercise.

A disturbance of glycogen metabolism at the level of *phosphohexose isomerase* [7] has been suggested in two adult brothers with muscle cramps and weakness after exercise and no rise of venous lactate after ischaemic exercise. The same defect was found in an adult with weakness and fatigability of the muscles of the face and extremities [5].

Based on histochemical findings, an 8-year-old boy, with muscle cramps after exercise, was thought to suffer from *phosphorylase b kinase* deficiency [9].

Finally, there are glycogenoses in which more than one enzyme seems to be lacking, or in which detailed in vitro and vivo studies fail to reveal any enzymatic defect of glycogen metabolism [2,3,8].

In none of these diseases is treatment satisfactory, despite the fact that in many glycogen storage diseases the specific biochemical abnormality is known [6].

References   1   Huying,F.,Fernandes,J.
X-chromosomal inheritance of liver glycogenosis with
phosphorylase kinase deficiency.
Amer.J.hum.Genet.1969,21:275–284

2   Larsson,L.-E.,Linderholm,H.,Müller,R.,Ringqvist,T.,Sörnäs,R.
Hereditary metabolic myopathy with paroxymal
myoglobinuria due to abnormal glycolysis.
J.Neurol.Neurosurg.Psychiat.1964,27:361–380

3   Linderholm,H.,Müller,R.,Ringqvist,T.,Sörnäs,R.
Hereditary abnormal muscle metabolism with hyperkinetic
circulation during exercise.
Acta med.scand.1969,185:153–166

4 Migeon,B.R.,Huying,F.
Glycogen-storage disease associated with phosphorylase kinase deficiency: evidence for X inactivation.
Amer.J.hum.Genet.1974,26:360–368

5 Mrozek,K.,Niebrój-Dobosz,I.,Lazarowicz,J.
Glycogen myopathy with a probable deficiency of phosphohexose isomerase.
Neurol.Neurochir.pol.1973,23:267–271

6 Rowland,L.P.,DiMauro,S.,Bank,W.J.
Glycogen storage disease of muscle. Problems in biochemical genetics.
Birth Def.,Orig.Art.Ser.1971,7:43–51

7 Satoyoshi,E.,Kowa,H.
A myopathy due to glycolytic abnormality.
Arch.Neurol.(Chic.)1967,17:248–256

8 Slotwiner,P.,Song,S.K.,Maker,H.S.
Myopathy resembling McArdle's syndrome.
Arch.Neurol.(Chic.)1969,20:586–598

9 Strugalska-Cynowska,M.
Disturbances in the activity of phosphorylase b kinase in a case of McArdle myopathy.
Folia histochem.cytochem.1967,5:151–156

10 Thomson,W.H.S.,MacLaurin,J.C.,Prineas,J.W.
Skeletal muscle glycogenosis: an investigation of two dissimilar cases.
J.Neurol.Neurosurg.Psychiat.1963,26:60–68

Acid maltase deficiency or type II glycogenosis, is an inborn error of glycogen metabolism due to deficiency of lysosomal acid maltase (acid alpha-1,4-glucosidase).

Infantile type (Pompe's disease)

The infantile type manifests itself a few months after birth with generalized muscular weakness, marked hypotonia, cardiomegaly and hepatomegaly. Dyspnoea, cyanosis, poor sucking and weak crying are the presenting findings. In addition, enlargement of the tongue and psychomotor retardation may occur.

The electrocardiogram shows a short PR interval and high voltage QRS complexes [12].

There is a generalized glycogen storage in the skeletal muscles, the heart, the central nervous system [9], the peripheral nerves [1] and various other organs, especially the liver. Storage of a non-glycogen polysaccharide [14] and metachromatic material [10] is also sometimes found in the skeletal muscles.

Involvement of the anterior horn cells of the spinal cord, the peripheral nerves and the skeletal muscles may together give rise to severe motor symptoms.

The prognosis of this type is unfavourable and most patients die within the first year of life.

The enzyme deficiency can be demonstrated biochemically and histochemically [3] in the muscle tissue.

Childhood type

When the glycogenosis is less generalized, especially when there is no enlargement of the heart and the liver, the survival time is much longer.
These patients show a mild proximal myopathy and were diagnosed in the past as limb-girdle dystrophy.
The clinical picture and the progression of this childhood type are very variable.

Adult type

These patients suffer from a slowly progressive myopathy with onset in adult life. The proximal muscles are more involved than the distal ones and the muscles of the pelvic girdle more so than those of the shoulder girdle [7]. Respiratory muscle involvement may also occur.
As a rule the serum creatine phosphokinase activity is increased. In blood smears vacuolated lymphocytes may be seen. Liver function tests are usually within normal limits.
As in the other types, electromyography of the paretic muscles may show motor unit potentials of short duration, and also abnormal irritability consisting of fibrillation potentials, short positive waves, and high frequency and myotonic discharges without clinical signs of myotonia [4,7]. In adults, the myotonic discharges are mainly found in the paraspinal muscles. Motor nerve conduction velocities are normal. The electrocardiogram is normal.
Muscle biopsy shows a variation in the diameter of the muscle fibres and an increased number of internal nuclei. The presence of vacuoles in the muscle fibres is of diagnostic importance; they are usually multiple and very small. The number found in a given biopsy may vary considerably,

and occasionally may be found in only a few fibres. The greater number of vacuoles contain PAS-positive granules and also show a very high activity of acid phosphatase. This histochemical finding is highly suggestive of acid maltase deficiency. Electron microscopy shows an accumulation of glycogen lying not only freely between the myofilaments but also in membrane-bound sacs and in autophagic vacuoles [4]. Various mito- chondrial abnormalities may also be seen [5].

Cultured muscle fibres from a biopsy of a patient with adult-onset acid maltase deficiency demonstrated the same morphologic and biochemical abnormalities characteristic of the biopsied muscle, supporting the concept of a biochemically distinct primary myopathy in man [2].

The enzyme deficiency can be demonstrated by biochemical assay of the muscle tissue. There is an excess of muscle glycogen, but this may vary con- siderably from case to case and in different muscles in the same patient.

Acid maltase deficiency is also present in liver biopsies but there is no significant glycogen excess.

The ratio acid maltase (maximal activity at pH 4.5–5.0) to neutral maltase (optimal activity at pH 6.5) of the leukocytes is lowered. When instead of maltose, glycogen is used as the in vitro substrate, the diagnosis can be made by estimation of this ratio in isolated leukocytes at pH 4 [9].

There is a marked decrease of urinary acid maltase excretion in adult acid maltase deficiency. Neutral maltase is unchanged and this is reflected by a shift of optimum pH towards the neutral range. As a result the ratio of urinary acid to neutral maltase activity is decreased [13].

There is an autosomal recessive inheritance in all types. In the 14th–16th week of pregnancy prenatal diagnosis of the infantile type is possible by amniocentesis and fluid cell culture [8].

Acid maltase deficiency carriers can be detected by assay of the enzyme in muscle biopsies [6]. The activity of muscle acid maltase of the heter- ozygotes may be only slightly lower than the lowest activity of normal controls.

Analysis of the maltase system in urine shows a decrease of daily urinary excretion of acid maltase and a decrease of the acid to neutral activity ratio. Therefore, urinary enzyme assay seems a simple and reliable method for the detection of heterozygotes [13].

References   1   Araoz,C.,Sun,C.N.,Shenefelt,R.,White,H.J.
Glycogenosis type II (Pompe's disease): ultrastructure of peripheral nerves.
Neurology(Minneap.)1974,24:739–742

2   Askanas,V.,Engel,W.K.,DiMauro,S.,Brooks,B.R.,Mehler,M.
Adult-onset acid maltase deficiency. Morphologic and biochemical abnormalities reproduced in cultured muscle.
New Engl.J.Med.1976,294:573–578

3   Cardiff,R.D.
A histochemical and electron microscopic study of skeletal muscle in a case of Pompe's disease (glycogenosis II).
Pediatrics 1966,37:249–259

4   Engel,A.G.
Acid maltase deficiency in adults: studies in four cases of a syndrome which may mimic muscular dystrophy or other myopathies.
Brain 1970,93:599–606

5   Engel,A.G.,Dale,A.J.D.
Autophagic glycogenosis of late onset with mitochondrial abnormalities: light and electron microscopic observations.
Proc.Mayo Clin.1968,43:233–279

6   Engel,A.G.,Gomez,M.R.
Acid maltase levels in muscle in heterozygous acid maltase deficiency and in non-weak and neuromuscular disease controls.
J.Neurol.Neurosurg.Psychiat.1970,33:801–804

7   Engel,A.G.,Gomez,M.R.,Seybold,M.E.,Lambert,E.H.
The spectrum and diagnosis of acid maltase deficiency.
Neurology(Minneap.)1973,23:95–106

8   Galjaard,H.,Mekes,M.,DeJosselinDeJong,J.E.,Niermeyer,M.F.
A method for rapid prenatal diagnosis of glycogenosis II (Pompe's disease).
Clin.Chim.Acta 1973,49:361–375

9   Hogan,G.R.,Gutmann,L.,Schmidt,R.,Gilbert,E.
Pompe's disease.
Neurology(Minneap.)1969,19:894–900

10   Hudgson,P.,Fulthorpe,J.J.
The pathology of type II skeletal muscle glycogenosis.
J.Path.1975,116:139–147

11   Koster,J.F.,Slee,R.G.,Hülsmann,W.C.
The use of leucocytes as an aid in the diagnosis of glycogen
storage disease type II (Pompe's disease).
Clin.chim.Acta 1974,51:319–325

12   Lenard,H.G.,Schaub,J.,Keutel,J.,Osang,M.
Electromyography in type II glycogenosis.
Neuropädiatrie 1974,5:410–424

13   Mehler,M.,DiMauro,S.
Late-onset acid maltase deficiency. Detection of patients
and heterozygotes by urinary enzyme assay.
Arch.Neurol.(Chic.)1976,33:692–695

14   Wolfe,H.,Cohen,R.B.
Non-glycogen polysaccharide storage in glycogenosis type 2
(Pompe's disease).
Arch.Path.1968,86:579–584

Amylo-1,6-glucosidase, or the debranching enzyme, makes the inner structure of glycogen accessible to phosphorylase action by splitting the alpha-1,6 linkages at the branch points. In the absence of this enzyme only the outer straight chains of glycogen can be broken down by phosphorylase. This results in an accumulation of glycogen with short outer chains (limit dextrin). Amylo-1,6-glucosidase deficiency, therefore, is also called limit dextrinosis. The disease has also been named after Forbes (1953) and after Cori (1956) and is termed type III glycogenosis according to the classification by Cori.

In young children the disease can manifest with psychomotor retardation and hepatomegaly. There is often an increased susceptibility to infection. When there is clinical affection of the skeletal muscles, the infants show hypotonia and weakness.
The enlargement of the liver may disappear with age; the patient by then may have virtually no complaints, notwithstanding the persistence of the underlying enzymatic defect.

After short reports were published [2,4] in which adults suffering from the disease were mentioned, full descriptions of two adult patients were given [1,3].
These patients had a history of enlargement of the liver during childhood. They also complained from childhood of early muscle fatigue and muscle stiffness after strenuous exercise, such as climbing stairs or running. No changes in muscle tone or strength were observed [3], but one patient showed marked wasting of the intrinsic muscles of the hands [1].
It is of interest that both reports mention an elevated level of serum uric acid, one patient showing swelling, slight pain and redness at the metatarsophalangeal joint of the left great toe, the other aching and mild swelling of the fingers.
Serum creatine phosphokinase activity was increased.
No rise of venous lactate was seen after ischaemic forearm exercise.
Electromyographic studies revealed moderately increased insertional activ-

ity, brief pseudomyotonic discharges, abundant fibrillations and sharp positive potentials at rest [1].

In patients with amylo-1,6-glucosidase deficiency there is a rise of blood lactate after oral administration of glucose. Intravenous administration of glucagon after an overnight fast is not followed by an elevation of blood glucose. The response of blood glucose to epinephrine is absent or diminished.

Muscle biopsy shows excessive deposition of PAS-positive material, especially in the subsarcolemmal regions.

Electron microscopy reveals abnormal accumulation of glycogen, mainly subsarcolemmal and intermyofibrillar. The ultrastructural features of the glycogen granules seem to be normal, but biochemical testing reveals that the glycogen is structurally abnormal and has short outer straight chains. On biochemical assay there is a marked increase of glycogen content in the muscle and in the liver. Also, in some cases, the erythrocyte glycogen was found to be raised.

Diagnosis can be made by demonstration of the enzyme deficiency in the leukocytes [5,6], the muscle or the liver.

There is an autosomal recessive type of inheritance. A low level of the debranching enzyme activity was found in the leukocytes of the parents of a patient [6], suggesting that this enzyme assay may be useful in the detection of the heterozygote state.

References   1   Brunberg,J.A.,McCormick,W.F.,SchochetJr,S.S.
                       Type III glycogenosis. An adult with diffuse weakness and
                       muscle wasting.
                       Arch.Neurol.(Chic.)1971,25:171–178
                 2   HatcherJr,M.A.,SidburyJr,J.B.,Heyman,A.
                       Muscle glycogenosis in adults – A comparison of type III,
                       Forbes' disease, with type V, McArdle's disease.
                       Neurology(Minneap.)1964,14:255

3 Murase,T.,Ikeda,H.,Muro,T.,Nakao,K.,Sugita,H.
Myopathy associated with type III glycogenosis.
J.neurol.Sci.1973,20:287–295

4 Oliner,L.,Schulman,M.,Larner,J.
Myopathy associated with glycogen deposition resulting
from generalized lack of amylo-1,6-glucosidase.
Clin.Res.1961,9:243

5 Steinitz,K.,Bodur,H.,Arman,T.
Amylo-1,6-glucosidase activity in leucocytes from patients
with glycogen storage disease.
Clin.chim.Acta 1963,8:807–809

6 Williams,H.E.,Kendig,E.M.,Field,J.B.
Leukocyte debranching enzyme in glycogen storage disease.
J.clin.Invest.1963,42:656–660

Amylo-1,4 → 1,6-transglucosidase, or branching enzyme deficiency, is also named after Dorothy Andersen (1952, 1956) who first described the disorder.

The disease is type IV glycogenosis in the classification by Cori, and is sometimes called amylopectinosis because of the storage of an amylopectin-like polysaccharide.

The first demonstration of the postulated enzyme defect was given by Brown and Brown [2]. There is widespread storage of a polysaccharide with long outer chains and relatively few branch points. It has been suggested that the branched polysaccharide is synthesized via the reversible action of the debranching system [6].

All definite cases have been children who died within the first 4 years of life. In the original patient [1] there was glycogen storage in the liver, spleen and lymph nodes, while no abnormalities were found in the muscles. The second patient described [9], had atrophic extremities and hypotonic muscles. Post-mortem studies showed widespread deposition of abnormal polysaccharide, for instance, in the spinal cord, the heart and the skeletal muscles.

Another patient [4] had paretic muscles of the legs with absent tendon reflexes and contractures of both elbows and thumbs, probably of myogenic origin. His brother [3] had poor muscle tone and decreased tendon reflexes. Autopsy in both cases showed deposition of abnormal glycogen scattered in the skeletal muscles.

Marked muscular atrophy and weakness, absent tendon reflexes, bilateral congenital hip dislocation and contractures of the shoulder joints were described [8] in a patient with polysaccharide deposits in the skeletal muscles. The stored material stained blue with hematoxylin—eosin and alcian blue, and red with Best's carmine and the PAS reaction [7].

During life the diagnosis can be made by the demonstration of the enzyme deficiency and the abnormal glycogen in the leukocytes [3].

A cardio-skeletal myopathy presenting in adult life, with generalized muscle wasting and weakness, and deposition of material with the staining properties of the polysaccharide seen in branching enzyme deficiency [5], was not biochemically examined and therefore cannot be considered as a definite case.

No detailed chemical studies of glycogen structure or metabolism could be performed in a 78-year-old woman with slowly progressive muscle weakness, tremor and dementia. This patient also showed storage of material in the muscles with similar histochemical characteristics as those seen in branching enzyme deficiency [10].

References   1   Andersen,D.H.
Familial cirrhosis of the liver with storage of abnormal glycogen.
Lab.Invest.1956,5:11–20

2   Brown,B.I.,Brown,D.H.
Lack of an α-1,4-glucan: α-1,4-glucan-6-glycosyl transferase
in a case of type IV glycogenosis.
Proc.nat.Acad.Sci.USA1966,56:725–729

3   Fernandes,J.,Huying,F.
Branching enzyme-deficiency glycogenosis: studies
in therapy.
Arch.Dis.Childh.1968,43:347–352

4   Holleman,L.W.J.,VanderHaar,J.A.,DeVaan,G.A.M.
Type IV glycogenosis.
Lab.Invest.1966,15:357–367

5   Holmes,J.M.,Houghton,C.R.,Woolf,A.L.
A myopathy presenting in adult life with features suggestive
of glycogen storage disease.
J.Neurol.Neurosurg.Psychiat.1960,23:302–311

6   Huying,F.,Lee,E.Y.C.,Carter,J.H.,Welan,W.J.
Branching action of amylo-1,6-glucosidase/
oligo-1,4 → 1,4-glucantransferase.
FEBS Lett.1970,7:251–253

7   SchochetJr,S.S.,McCormick,W.F.,Kovarsky,J.
Light and electron microscopy of skeletal muscle in type IV
glycogenosis.
Acta Neuropath.1971,19:137–144

8   SchochetJr,S.S.,McCormick,W.F.,Zellweger,H.
Type IV glycogenosis (amylopectinosis). Light and electron
microscopic observations.
Arch.Path.1970,90:354–363

9   SidburyJr,J.B.,Mason,J.,BurnsJr,W.B.,Ruebner,B.H.
Type IV glycogenosis. Report of a case proven by
characterization of glycogen and studies at necropsy.
Bull.Johns Hopk.Hosp.1962,111:157–181

10   Torvik,A.,Dietrichson,P.,Svaar,H.,Hudgson,P.
Myopathy with tremor and dementia: a metabolic disorder?
Case report with postmortem study.
J.neurol.Sci.1974,21:181–190

Muscle phosphorylase deficiency is often called McArdle's disease and is considered as type V glycogenosis.

In 1951 McArdle described a myopathy due to a defect in muscle glycogen breakdown [5]. The enzymatic defect in glycogenolysis was found in 1959 and proved to be a deficiency of muscle phosphorylase [6,13].

Immunological studies failed to reveal an altered protein molecule corresponding to an enzymatically deficient phosphorylase [10]. The lack of phosphorylase is confined to skeletal muscle: phosphorylase activity is normal in the liver, leukocytes and erythrocytes.

Muscle glycogen content is usually increased but may be found to be normal. There is no abnormality of the glycogen structure.

The first symptoms may start in early childhood and consist of easy muscle fatigability. Some patients may have a history of occasional myoglobinuria. Acute renal failure associated with myoglobinuria has also been described [1,4].

In early adult life there is limitation of exercise due to cramping muscle pain which responds to rest. The cramps may last several hours after moderate exercise. The exercise intolerance may vary considerably from one patient to another or in the same patient.

In one patient symptoms developed after isometric rather than after isotonic exercise [11]. It is often possible for the patient to walk during long periods on level ground, but walking on grades or climbing stairs is soon followed by cramps in the muscles of the lower extremities. By intensive use of other muscles (hands, arms, jaws) painful cramps also occur in these muscles. There is no relation between the cramps and cold temperature, heavy meals, alcohol ingestion or sleep. Extreme fatigue and weakness of the exercising muscles may disappear completely within one minute when the patient is able to sustain non-strenuous exercise. This phenomenon has been named 'second wind' [7]. It is dependent on the availability of blood free fatty acids to the muscles, and has been explained by augmented or altered distribution of blood flow to the muscles [8].

Severe muscle cramps are occasionally followed by transient myoglobinuria. The interval between cramps and myoglobulinuria varies from less than an hour to several hours. The duration of myoglobulinuria seldom exceeds 48 hours.

Between attacks physical examination shows nothing abnormal.

After the fourth decade myoglobinuria tends to become very rare. At that time a persistent and progressive proximal muscle weakness may develop, especially in those patients who have been suffering from many severe attacks of myoglobinuria.

Ischaemic forearm exercise results within one minute in rapid fatigue and painful contracture of the flexor muscles. Wrist and fingers are flexed and cannot be stretched, either actively or passively. After the circulation is restored it may even take one to several hours before the situation gradually returns to normal.

Electromyography shows no electric activity of the maximal shortened muscle (true contracture). Contracture can also be induced by supra-maximal stimulation of the ulnar nerve, action potentials being recorded from the interosseus primus muscle.

The metabolic events that give rise to this contracture are unknown. After ischaemic forearm exercise there is no increase of venous lactate and pyruvate concentration. This lack of lactate response is very important in diagnosing McArdle's disease but is in no way specific for this disease. The same phenomenon may be seen in patients suffering from amylo-1,6-glucosidase deficiency (page 196), phosphofructokinase deficiency (page 206) and other diseases in which a block in the glycolytic pathway is suspected [12].

Light microscopy of a muscle biopsy shows subsarcolemmal blebs, often containing PAS-positive granules. The absence of total phosphorylase can also be seen by enzymhistochemistry. In a variant of the disease, phospho-rylase was found to be absent in a biopsy of one quadriceps muscle and appeared to be only decreased in the other quadriceps [9].

Ultrastructural studies showed that the glycogen accumulation occurs primarily under the sarcolemma and also in the intermyofibrillar space and between the thin filaments at the level of the I band [14].

Many studies have suggested that the disease has an autosomal recessive mode of inheritance [2]. However, it may well be that several genetic defects can lead to muscle phosphorylase deficiency.

A familial late-onset type of skeletal muscle phosphorylase deficiency was described by Engel, Eyerman and Williams [3] in a sister and brother.
The onset was at the age of 49 years in both patients. The woman showed severe muscular weakness and wasting, without muscular cramps. There was no muscle phosphorylase activity on quantitative biochemical assay. The man had painful cramps a few hours after exercise, without weakness. Total muscle phosphorylase activity was 35 per cent of normal. After ischaemic forearm exercise there was no rise of the lactate level in the sister and a normal elevation in the brother.

References   1   Bank,W.J.,DiMauro,S.,Rowland,L.P.
Renal failure in McArdle's disease.
New Engl.J.Med.1972,287:1102

2   Cochrane,P.,Hughes,R.R.,Buxton,P.H.,Yorke,R.A.
Myophosphorylase deficiency (McArdle's disease) in two interrelated families.
J.Neurol.Neurosurg.Psychiat.1973,36:217–224

3   Engel,W.K.,Eyerman,E.L.,Williams,H.E.
Late-onset type of skeletal-muscle phosphorylase deficiency.
A new familial variety with completely and partially affected subjects.
New Engl.J.Med.1963,268:135–137

4   Grünfeld,J.-P.,Ganeval,D.,Chanard,J.,Fardeau,M.,Dreyfus,J.C.
Acute renal failure in McArdle's disease.
New Engl.J.Med.1972,286:1237–1241

5   McArdle,B.
Myopathy due to defect in muscle glycogen breakdown.
Clin.Sci.1951,10:13–33

6   Mommaerts,W.F.H.M.,Illingworth,B.,Pearson,C.M.,Guillory,R.J.,Seraydarian,K.
A functional disorder of muscle associated with the absence of phosphorylase.

Proc.nat.Acad.Sci.USA1959,45:791–797

7   Pearson,C.M.,Rimer,D.G.,Mommaerts,W.F.H.M.
     A metabolic myopathy due to absence of muscle
     phosphorylase.
     Amer.J.Med.1961,30:502–517

8   Pernow,B.B.,Havel,R.J.,Jennings,D.B.
     The second wind phenomenon in McArdle's syndrome.
     Acta med.scand.(Suppl.)1967,142:294–307

9   Roelofs,R.I.,Corbin,J.,Peter,J.B.,Infante,E.
     A new variant of McArdle's disease.
     Neurology(Minneap.)1974,24:397

10   Rowland,L.P.,Fahn,S.,Schotland,D.L.
     McArdle's disease. Hereditary myopathy due to absence
     of muscle phosphorylase.
     Arch.Neurol.(Chic.)1963,9:325–342

11   Sahn,L.,Magee,K.R.
     Phosphorylase deficiency associated with isometric exercise
     intolerance.
     Neurology(Minneap.)1976,26:896–898.

12   Satoyoshi,E.,Kowa,H.
     A myopathy due to glycolytic abnormality.
     Arch.Neurol.(Chic.)1967,17:248–256

13   Schmid,R.,Mahler,R.
     Syndrome of muscular dystrophy with myoglobinuria:
     demonstration of a glycogenolytic defect in muscle.
     J.clin.Invest.1959,38:1040.

14   Schotland,D.L.,Spiro,D.,Rowland,L.P.,Carmel,P.
     Ultrastructural studies of muscle in McArdle's disease.
     (Deficiency of muscle phosphorylase).
     J.Neuropath.exp.Neurol.1965,24:629–644

Phosphofructokinase catalyzes the conversion of fructose-6-phosphate to fructose-1,6-diphosphate.

The deficiency of this enzyme in human skeletal muscle was first described in 1965 by Tarui, Okuno, Ikura, Tanaka, Suda and Nishikawa [5].

Because of the block in the Embden-Meyerhof pathway of glycolysis, there is an accumulation of muscle glycogen and hence the disease has also been called type VII glycogenosis.

From early childhood the patients suffer from exercise intolerance with painful muscle cramps — often accompanied by nausea — and occasionally followed by myoglobinuria. Between these episodes no signs are present on physical examination. Serum creatine phosphokinase activity is moderately increased. As in McArdle's disease (page 202) there is no rise of venous lactate after ischaemic forearm exercise. During this procedure a contracture of the flexor muscles of the forearm develops.

The patient described by Serratrice, Monges, Roux, Aquaron and Gambarelli [4] did not complain about muscle cramps or pigmenturia after exercise but showed a scapulo-peroneal myopathy.

Biopsy findings consist of variation in fibre diameter, subsarcolemmal accumulation of PAS-positive material and occasional necrotic fibres [6]. The absence of phosphofructokinase in the muscle fibres can also be demonstrated histochemically [1].

Immunological studies with antibody to purified normal human muscle phosphofructokinase showed that no enzymatically inactive form of phosphofructokinase was present in the patient's muscle [3]. The phosphofructokinase activity is normal in the leukocytes and is reduced to 50 per cent in the erythrocytes. It is suggested that human muscle phosphofructokinase is composed of one (M) sub-unit, while two non-identical sub-units (M and R) of the enzyme are present in erythrocytes [2]. When it is assumed that there is only a genetic lack of the M sub-unit in the disease, the 50 per cent residual enzyme activity in erythrocytes can be explained. Erythrocyte phosphofructokinase reduction can also be found in the parents of the patients [3], suggesting autosomal recessive inheritance.

References 1 Bonilla,E.,Schotland,D.L.
Histochemical diagnosis of muscle phosphofructokinase
deficiency.
Arch.Neurol(Chic.)1970,22:8–12

2 Layzer,R.B.,Rasmussen,J.
The molecular basis of muscle phosphofructokinase deficiency.
Arch.Neurol.(Chic.)1974,31:411–417

3 Layzer,R.B.,Rowland,L.P.,Ranney,H.M.
Muscle phosphofructokinase deficiency.
Arch.Neurol.(Chic.)1967,17:512–523

4 Serratrice,G.,Monges,A.,Roux,H.,Aquaron,R.,Gambarelli,D.
Forme myopathique du déficit en phosphofructokinase.
Rev.Neurol.1969,120:271–277

5 Tarui,S.,Okuno,G.,Ikura,Y.,Tanaka,T.,Suda,M.,Nishikawa,M.
Phosphofructokinase deficiency in skeletal muscle.
A new type of glycogenosis.
Biochem.biophys.Res.Commun.1965,19:517–523

6 Tobin,W.E.,Huijing,F.,Porro,R.S.,Salzman,R.T.
Muscle phosphofructokinase deficiency.
Arch.Neurol.(Chic.)1973,28:128–130

Other storage diseases

Storage of polysaccharides, other than glycogen, in the muscle tissue has occasionally been reported [1–3].

Proximal muscle weakness was seen in all cases, while two patients suffered from cardiomyopathy [1,2]. The muscle biopsies showed marked accumulation of PAS-positive material. In one case [2] the storaged material was only present in the type II fibres and was considered to be a glycoprotein.

Electron microscopy revealed that the material contained two components of different electron density. Biochemical analysis of the muscle tissue showed low glycogen content and an increased amount of a cetylpyridium chloride (CPC)-precipitable glycosaminoglycan-like material, which contained low (1 per cent) hexosamine, 10 per cent hexoses and 10 per cent proteins.

In another case [3] the storaged material was seen in both fibre types. Chemical analysis of the muscle tissue disclosed low glycogen content and an increased amount of CPC-precipitable glycosaminoglycans, containing 6.7 per cent hexosamine, 12.2 per cent hexoses and a small amount (5.2 per cent) of proteins.

If was suggested that the basic effect consisted of an excessive synthesis of the PAS-positive material.

References 1 Holmes,J.M.,Houghton,C.R.,Woolf,A.L.
               A myopathy presenting in adult life with features suggestive
               of glycogen storage disease.
               J.Neurol.Neurosurg.Psychiat.1960,23:302–311
            2 Karpati,G.,Carpenter,S.,Wolfe,L.S.,Sherwin,A.
               A peculiar polysaccharide accumulation in muscle in a case
               of cardioskeletal myopathy.
               Neurology(Minneap.)1969,19:553–564
            3 Radu,H.,Ionescu,V.,Georgescu,M.,Radu,A.
               A new metabolic disorder: myopathy with
               glycosamino(sialo)glycans accumulation.
               Europ.Neurol.1974,12:209–225

Disorders of muscle lipid metabolism

The only disorder of muscle lipid metabolism known to be due to an enzyme deficiency, is carnitine palmityl transferase deficiency (page 219). In this disease there is no lipid excess in the muscle fibres.

There is also a heterogenous group of disorders that have in common the excess amount of lipid droplets in the muscle fibres. These disorders are referred to as lipid storage diseases (pages 212 and 215).

It has been suggested that the abnormal accumulation of lipid may be a consequence of a defect in any of the enzymes participating in the oxidative catabolism of fatty acids, or may be the result of an uncontrolled synthesis of fatty acids or of a block in the lipolytic release of fatty acids from triglycerides [1]. Only in muscle carnitine deficiency (page 212) is the defect of the lipid metabolism known, although there may be different causes for this deficiency.

In other cases of lipid storage in muscle the responsible metabolic defect remained unidentified.

Excess lipid accumulation is also frequently present in many cases of the so-called 'mitochondrial myopathies' (page 121) and in fact the two groups of muscular disorders do overlap.

Reference   1   Engel,A.G.,Siekert,R.G.
Lipid storage myopathy responsive to prednisone.
Arch.Neurol.(Chic.)1972,27:174–181

Carnitine (gamma-trimethylamino-beta-hydroxybutyrate) is important for the transport of long-chain fatty acids into mitochondria where they can undergo beta-oxidation.

It is found in high concentration in normal human skeletal muscle.

The first case of muscle carnitine deficiency was described in 1973 by Engel and Angelini [3]. Subsequent reports showed that defective carnitine transport across cell membranes may be more wide-spread, and not be limited to muscle alone. Consequently there may be impaired liver function, cardiac involvement [7] and abnormalities in the leukocytes and Schwann cells [6].

The first symptoms become evident in early infancy [7], but can also develop in childhood [1,5] or in middle life [6]. There is a progressive and generalized muscular weakness, especially of the limb-girdles. Often the cranial muscles are paretic.

When there is also involvement of the peripheral nerves additional symptoms of a neuropathy may develop: weakness of distal muscles, neurogenic electromyographic findings and decrease in nerve conduction velocities.

The activity of serum creatine phosphokinase was slightly or moderately elevated. Serum carnitine levels were normal [1,6,7] or low [4,5]. Liver carnitine levels were normal [4] or abnormally low [5]. Carnitine palmityl transferase activity in muscle tissue was normal [2,3].

In vivo, forearm metabolic studies showed impaired utilization of long-chain fatty acids and a compensatory increased glucose uptake by muscle [5]. During a brief fast, there was a marked inappropriate rise in plasma free fatty acids and ketones, resulting in a profound keton-acidosis [2].

Muscle biopsies showed a variation in muscle fibre diameter and an increase of internal nuclei. The most characteristic finding was the presence of numerous small vacuoles, predominantly affecting the type I fibres. These vacuoles were filled with lipid droplets, as was readily seen with the Oil red O staining method.

Ultrastructurally the vacuoles were lacking limiting membranes. They were empty or contained low electron dense material. The vacuoles were often present in long parallel rows, could cause disruption of the myofibrillar architecture and were adjacent to abnormally shaped mitochondria.

The cause of carnitine deficiency is unknown, but the pathogenesis may differ in the patients described so far.
Prednisone therapy had a beneficial effect on the muscle weakness, but the muscle carnitine level was not influenced by this drug [4]. The oral administration of DL-carnitine in combination with a medium-chain tri-glyceride diet also resulted in improvement of exercise tolerance and muscle strength [1,5].
Again, this kind of therapy had no influence on the muscle carnitine level, and the liver carnitine level also remained unchanged.

An autosomal recessive inheritance is suspected. Thus far the asymptomatic parents of only one patient were examined [7], and they showed abnormally low muscle carnitine levels. Therefore, the assay of muscle carnitine may be an important method of recognizing the heterozygote state.

References   1   Angelini,C.,Lücke,S.,Cantarutti,F.
                       Carnitine deficiency of skeletal muscle: report of a treated
                       case.
                       Neurology(Minneap.)1976,26:633–637
                2   Bank,W.J.,Schotland,D.L.,Capuzzi,D.M.,Morrison,A.D.
                       Muscle carnitine deficiency, fat mobilization and ketoacidosis.
                       J.Neuropath.exp.Neurol.1976,35:373
                3   Engel,A.G.,Angelini,C.
                       Carnitine deficiency of human skeletal muscle with associated
                       lipid storage myopathy: a new syndrome.
                       Science 1973,179:899–902
                4   Engel,A.G.,Angelini,C.,Nelson,R.A.
                       Identification of carnitine deficiency as a cause of human
                       lipid storage myopathy.
                       In:Exploratory Concepts in Muscular Dystrophy II.

Proceedings of an International Conference,Carefree,Ariz.,
October15–19,1973.Amsterdam,Excerpta Medica,
pp.601–617.(Int.Congr.Ser.333).

5   Karpati,G.,Carpenter,S.,Engel,A.G.,Watters,G.,Allen,J.,
Rothman,S.,Klassen,G.,Mamer,A.
The syndrome of systemic carnitine deficiency.
Clinical, morphologic, biochemical, and pathophysiologic
features.
Neurology(Minneap.)1975,25:16–24

6   Markesbery,W.R.,McQuillen,M.P.,Procopis,P.G.,
Harrison,A.R.,Engel,A.G.
Muscle carnitine deficiency. Association with lipid myopathy,
vacuolar neuropathy, and vacuolated leucocytes.
Arch.Neurol.(Chic.)1974,31:320–324

7   Vandyke,D.H.,Griggs,R.C.,Markesbery,W.,DiMauro,S.
Hereditary carnitine deficiency of muscle.
Neurology(Minneap.)1975,25:154–159

In 1969 Bradley, Hudgson, Gardner-Medwin and Walton [2] published a preliminary report on a patient suffering from a myopathy associated with greatly increased amounts of sarcoplasmic lipid. In 1973 a complete communication was given on the same patient, a 23-year-old woman with parents who were first cousins. She had suffered two attacks of proximal muscle weakness which remitted spontaneously. The first attack lasted a few weeks, the second $2\frac{1}{2}$ years. Muscular weakness without wasting was present in the limb girdles and neck muscles. Serum creatine phosphokinase activity was slightly raised. The electromyogram showed moderate increase of low-amplitude, short-duration motor unit potentials and polyphasic potentials. Motor nerve conduction velocity was normal.

The muscle triglyceride content was greatly increased, the fatty acid composition of the triglyceride was normal. Muscle tricaproin lipase activity was normal.

There was a very marked increase of neutral lipid droplets in the muscle fibres, especially in the type I fibres. A number of these fibres showed excessive activities of mitochondrial oxidative enzymes. Electron microscopy of several biopsies showed long strands of lipid droplets between the myofibrils. An increase of abnormally shaped mitochondria with amorphous electron-dense and paracrystalline ('parking-lot') inclusions, was also seen. However, the abnormality of lipid metabolism was considered to be the primary lesion in this case.

Since then other and similar cases have been described [6,7] with an impressive response to treatment with high doses of prednisone.

Coupling of oxidative phosphorylation by the isolated muscle mitochondria was normal [6].

A skeletal muscle disorder associated with intermittent symptoms and a possible defect of lipid metabolism was described in 1970 by Engel, Vick, Glueck and Levy [3].

The patients were identical twin 18-year-old girls, who at 4 or 5 years of age began to experience intermittent symptoms of painful muscle cramps, frequently but not always related to exercise several hours earlier. There was no weakness, but severe attacks were associated with myoglobinuria. Physical examination and detailed neurological examination did not reveal any abnormalities. There was a normal rise of blood lactate after ischaemic exercise. Electromyography was normal in three muscles and borderline neuropathic in another. Motor and sensory conduction times were normal. Light and electron microscopy of a muscle biopsy showed an excess number of lipid droplets, especially in the type I fibres.

Fasting for 24 to 60 hours or a isocaloric high-fat low-carbohydrate diet produced cramping muscle aches, general malaise and mild nausea. At the same time there was a marked rise of serum creatine phosphokinase, aldolase, GOT, GPT, and LDH activities.

In addition there was no rise of plasma and urine total ketone bodies, in contrast to a marked increase in normal controls.

During fasting the free fatty acid mobilization was normal. Refeeding with a normal diet corrected all the abnormal signs and symptoms within 12 hours.

Plasma and urinary ketone bodies were normally produced by oral ingestion of medium-chain-length triglycerides. A selective defect in the utilization of long-chain fatty acids was considered as a possible explanation for the clinical and laboratory findings in these patients.

Marked subsarcolemmal accumulation of lipid in both fibre types was reported in patients treated by adrenalectomy for Cushing's syndrome [8]. Excessive accumulation of lipid droplets, especially in the type I fibres, was also found in a 9-year-old boy with pyruvate decarboxylase deficiency [1], but this patient had episodes of ataxia and no history or symptoms of a myopathic disorder.

Congenital lipid storage diseases

A patient with a congenital non-progressive lipid storage disease had normal serum carnitine levels and normal muscle carnitine and carnitine palmityl transferase levels [5]. Muscle biopsy revealed type I fibre predominance and neutral fat droplets in both type I and type II fibres.

Another patient suffering from a congenital and morphologically regressive myopathy with generalized weakness, hepatomegaly and macroglossia showed not only an excess of lipid, especially in the type I fibres, but also mitochondrial and glycogen excess in the muscle fibres. The disease was called mitochondria-lipid-glycogen (MLG) disease of muscle [4].

References

1 Blass,J.P.,Kark,R.A.P.,Engel,W.K.
Clinical studies of a patient with pyruvate decarboxylase deficiency.
Arch.Neurol.(Chic.)1971,25:449–460.

2 Bradley,W.G.,Hudgson,P.,Gardner-Medwin,D.,Walton,J.N.
Myopathy associated with abnormal lipid metabolism in skeletal muscle.
Lancet 1969,I:495–498

3 Engel,W.K.,Vick,N.A.,Glueck,C.J.,Levy,R.I.
A skeletal-muscle disorder associated with intermittent symptoms and a possible defect of lipid metabolism.
New Engl.J.Med.1970,282:697–704

4 Jerusalem,F.,Angelini,C.,Engel,A.G.,Groover,R.V.
Mitochondria-lipid-glycogen (MLG) disease of muscle.
A morphologically regressive congenital myopathy.
Arch.Neurol.(Chic.)1973,29:162–169

5 Jerusalem,F.,Spiess,H.,Baumgartner,G.
Lipid storage myopathy with normal carnitine levels.
J.neurol.Sci.1975,24:273–282

6 Johnson,M.A.,Fulthorpe,J.J.,Hudgson,P.
Lipid storage myopathy: a recognizable clinico-pathological entity?
Acta neuropath.1973,24:97–106

7   Pinelli,P.,Poloni,M.,Nappi,G.,Scelsi,R.
     A case of late onset lipid storage myopathy.
     Electromyographic, histochemical and ultrastructural findings.
     Europ.Neurol.1975,13:273–284
8   Prineas,J.,Hall,R.,Barwick,D.D.,Watson,A.J.
     Myopathy associated with pigmentation following
     adrenalectomy for Cushing's syndrome.
     Quart.J.Med.1968,37:63–77

Carnitine palmityl transferase is an enzyme bound to the inner mitochondrial membrane. It plays a role in the esterification with carnitine of long-chain fatty acyl residues and serves the transport of activated fatty acids across the mitochondrial inner membrane to the site of β-oxidation.

In 1973 DiMauro and DiMauro [2] described a 29-year-old man with muscle carnitine palmityl transferase deficiency.

The findings in this patient and in his 33-year-old brother — who had identical symptoms — were described in more detail in 1975 [1].

The propositus had episodes of myoglobinuria from the age of 13 years that were not usually related to exercise. Occasionally he had stiffness of the muscles after prolonged exercise, but he never complained of painful cramps. Examination revealed no abnormalities between these episodes. The electromyogram was normal.

Serum creatine phosphokinase activity was within normal limits. Ischaemic exercise was followed by a normal rise of venous lactate and did not induce contracture.

Histochemical investigations showed no structural changes of the muscle fibres, and there was no evidence of lipid accumulation as judged by the Oil red 0 reaction. Ultrastructural studies revealed occasional rounded structures with low electron density, probably lipid, in type I fibres.

Biochemical investigations of the muscle tissue revealed a complete absence of carnitine palmityl transferase. In both patients the glycogen content was normal and the carnitine level was slightly raised.

The activities of muscle phosphorylase and phosphofructokinase were normal.

The outstanding abnormality in these patients was an increased content of plasma triglycerides and plasma free fatty acids. This was the result of the inadequate oxidation of long-chain free fatty acids by muscle due to the lack of carnitine palmityl transferase. There was an absence of plasma ketone production in response to 72-hour fasting. Oral ingestion of medium chain triglycerides resulted in a prompt, normal ketonaemia, suggesting that the oxidation of these fatty acids is independent of carnitine palmityl transferases, since in most tissue investigated, medium-chain fatty acids are activated at the same site of β-oxidation, viz. the mitochondrial matrix.

References   1   Bank,W.J.,DiMauro,S.,Bonilla,E.,Capuzzi,D.M.,Rowland,L.P.
                         A disorder of muscle lipid metabolism and myoglobinuria.
                         Absence of carnitine palmityl transferase.
                         New Engl.J.Med.1975,292:443–449
                   2   DiMauro,S.,DiMauro,P.M.M.
                         Muscle carnitine palmityltransferase deficiency and
                         myoglobinuria.
                         Science 1973,182:929–931

Polymyositis and dermatomyositis

The name polymyositis is applied to non-hereditary and inflammatory myo-pathies.

In the presence of a characteristic skin rash, the term dermatomyositis is used.

The age distribution suggests a bimodal curve [28], with a childhood peak (5–15 years of age) and an adult peak (45–55 years of age).

There are many classifications of these disorders [6,34,37,45], but due to their pleomorphic clinical presentation and the unknown aetiology or mechanisms of pathogenesis, any classification will necessarily be deficient. The Research Group on Neuromuscular Diseases of the World Federation of Neurology accepted the following classification [13]:

α *polymyositis* (possibly an organ-specific auto-immune disease), acute, subacute and chronic forms;

β *polymyositis or dermatomyositis* when occurring as one feature of what may prove to be a non-organ-specific auto-immune disease, including polymyositis associated with systemic lupus erythematosus, rheumatic fever, rheumatoid arthritis, progressive systemic sclerosis, polyarteritis nodosa, and polymyopathy in Sjögren's syndrome;

γ *polymyositis or dermatomyositis* occurring possibly as a conditioned auto-immune response in malignant disease.

Muscular manifestations

Symmetrical weakness of the proximal limb muscles and the neck flexors are the most characteristic clinical features. Dysphagia and dysphonia are also frequently present [37]. In the acute form, severe constitutional symptoms and widespread muscular pain and tenderness may be found. These features may be absent in the subacute and chronic forms. In the latter the proximal muscles of the lower limbs are usually first involved. In-volvement of the facial [4,38], and extraocular muscles [43] is rare.

The deep tendon reflexes are normal or slightly decreased.

Muscle atrophy does not occur until late in the course of the disease and tends to remain mild or moderate in extent. Also in later stages, muscular contractures and calcifications may develop. The latter can be detected by roentgenologic examination, in which case large masses may be seen [33].

Cutaneous manifestations

The dermatologic features consist of an erythematous eruption on the face. This rash is frequently in butterfly distribution, includes a lilac discolouration of the upper eyelids (heliotrope rash) and may be associated with periorbital oedema. In severe cases of dermatomyositis, erythema, a scaly rash or teleangiectasia can be seen on the forehad, the neck, shoulders, upper chest, back, knuckles, elbows, knees and medial malleoli. In the periungual area local vasculitis can be observed [23].

Late-stage dermatomyositis is characterized by calcification of the skin and subcutaneous tissue. Skin calcification is usually circumscribed and nodular, and tends to occur more frequently in children than in adults.

Other manifestations

Raynaud syndrome is a relatively frequent feature, especially in polymyositis or dermatomyositis with associated connective tissue diseases. The cyanosis or blanching is mainly seen in one or several fingers and to a lesser extent in the toes, especially as a result of general cooling.

Arthralgia is common, but is usually minimal and transitory. When more severe arthritis is present, the possibility of association with rheumatoid arthritis or systemic lupus erythematosus should be considered.

Pulmonary manifestations may be the presenting sign of polymyositis or dermatomyositis [9,41], or may occur later in the evolution of the disease. The predominant symptoms are non-productive cough and dyspnoea. The histopathologic picture consists of organizing and interstitial pneumonitis and bronchiolitis, which later progresses to interstitial fibrosis.

Cardiac arhythmias, heart block and electrocardiographic alterations have been reported in only a minority of cases.

Intestinal disorders have also been reported in some patients. In dermatomyositis in childhood, ulcerative lesions of the gastrointestinal tract may be present [3].

Hypomobility of the oesophagus may be an additional factor to the dysphagia that is caused by weakness of the pharyngeal musculature.

Laboratory findings

Serum creatine phosphokinase (CPK) activity may be raised and seems to be a more sensitive estimation than that of other serum enzyme activities, such as aldolase or glutamic oxalocetic transaminase. The degree of elevation of serum CPK activity does not correlate with the degree of weakness and disability [15,35].

In about 50 per cent of the cases the erythrocyte sedimentation rate is mildly raised [15,34]. Non-specific elevation of serum gamma-globulins has been reported.

Electromyography

Polyphasic, brief, small, abundant motor-unit action potentials are present, together with spontaneous fibrillations, positive sharp waves and increased insertional irritability. In addition bizarre high-frequency repetitive discharges with abrupt onset and termination, and of constant frequency and wave form, can be seen. This electromyographic phenomenon is indicative of increased muscle membrane irritability, and superficially resembles the myotonic response. It has formerly been referred to as 'pseudo-myotonic' discharges.

Motor nerve conduction velocities are normal.

Muscle pathology

The muscle biopsy may show no, or only minimal abnormalities [15,42,45], while cellular infiltrates may be absent [32].

The histopathological features most frequently seen include: (1) interstitial or perivascular infiltration with inflammatory cells, mainly lymphocytes and plasma cells; (2) abundant structural changes such as necrotic fibres with phagocytosis, basophilic fibres with vesicular nuclei and prominent nucleoli, and vacuolated fibres; (3) abnormalities in the size of both type I and type II fibres; (4) increase in the number of the fibres with internal nuclei; (5) increase of endomysial connective tissue.

Cytoplasmic bodies and rods may be seen in some muscle fibres [8].

Atrophy and necrosis of both fibre types in a perifascicular distribution should alert one to the diagnosis of polymyosistis or dermatomyositis – often in children – but it is only present in a relatively small number of the biopsies. Widespread necrotizing vasculitis is mainly present in childhood dermatomyositis [3,10].

In these cases ultrastructural studies revealed the primary occurrence of an angiopathy, represented by endothelial degeneration and regeneration, followed by thrombus formation and the infarction of the muscle tissue [2]. In adults, ultrastructural lesions are non-specific, and include focal degeneration of myofilaments, streaming of the Z discs, mitochondrial abnormalities, an increase of autophagocytic vacuoles, macrophages, lipid droplets and lysosomes [21,27].

The capillaries and venules show thickening and reduplications of the basement membranes. The inflammatory cells are small lymphocytes, enlarged activated lymphocytes and a few plasma cells and granulocytes. No abnormalities were observed in the end-plates and intramuscular nerve fibres.

Many investigators have observed intranuclear and intracytoplasmic virus-like inclusions: microtubules resembling the helical nucleocapsids of myxoviruses [11,21,40] and of paramyxoviruses [18,25,47] and spherical particles resembling picorna viruses, most likely of the Coxsackie group [12,26,27].

Association with neoplasia

Most authors agree that the association of neoplasia with polymyositis, and in particular with dermatomyositis, occurs too frequently to be accidental. The exact frequency of this association is very difficult to assess and varies from 5 to over 50 per cent in different series. No doubt there is a propensity for cases complicated by malignancy to be reported in the literature more frequently than uncomplicated cases [6,39]. Although the incidence of polymyositis with malignancy may be less than was previously thought, the association between dermatomyositis and neoplasia, particularly in males over the age of 40 years, seems to be present in a relatively high proportion of the cases [15]. All kind of tumors have been reported.

Carcinoma of the lung, breast, ovary, uterus and stomach were most frequently the primary sites, in addition to other malignancies such as sarcoma, leukaemia, malignant lymphoma and Hodgkin's disease.

In most cases the manifestations of dermatomyositis or polymyositis preceded those of the tumor. In some cases the tumor had not been found prior to post-mortem examination; and while treatment of the tumor may have a favourable effect on the associated muscular or skin lesions, there have been cases in which these manifestations appeared following the successful treatment of a tumor.

Aetiology and pathogenesis

The cause and pathogenesis of polymyositis and dermatomyositis are unknown, but viruses and cellular and humoral immunologic mechanisms may play a role.

The presence of virus-like particles, as seen by electron microscopy, has given rise to the possibility of a viral infection being the cause in some cases. However, there is only morphological evidence for such a viral theory. So far, no virus has been isolated and no epidemiologic evidence of a direct infectious agent has been found [28].

The auto-immune hypothesis has been put forward because of (a) the association of polymyositis and dermatomyositis with connective tissue disorders, (b) their response to treatment with corticosteroids or immuno-suppressive drugs, and (c) the fact that the onset is sometimes preceded by viral infections or the use of drugs, suggesting a mechanism of hypersensitivity. Other indications for the immunological theory are: lymphocytes from patients with polymyositis were cytotoxic to human fetal muscle cultures, while serum from these patients, or lymphocytes from those with other neuromuscular disorders, did not destroy the cultures [14]. Anti-lymphocytic antiserum appeared to prevent this cytotoxic action by lymphocytes.

Lymphotoxin, a mediator of delayed hypersensitivity, is produced by lymphocytes and by muscle from patients with dermatomyositis or polymyositis [22].

In muscle biopsies of patients with polymyositis and dermatomyositis, granular deposits of IgG, IgM and C3 were seen in the walls of the blood vessels, particularly in cases of childhood dermatomyositis [46]. This led to the hypothesis of immune-complex-induced vascular injury in these disorders.

In the context of the immunological pathogenesis, the demonstration of hereditary complement (C2) deficiency in a patient with dermatomyositis [24], and the report of X-linked agammaglobulinaemia in a patient with dermatomyositis and cerebral vasculitis [19], seem to be of importance.

Treatment

Beneficial effect can be obtained by treatment with corticosteroids.

Some authors start with daily high doses of prednisone, usually 50–100 mg in three daily doses, depending on the severity of the disease. This dose is reduced, in the course of about 3 months, to a maintenance dose usually of 5–20 mg per day, and continued for at least 2–5 years. Following this, an attempt should be made yearly to decrease the dosage gradually, in order to determine whether the disease still remains active.

Other authors recommended a 100 mg single dose daily for 3–4 weeks and gradual switching to a high, single dosage of prednisone every other day [16]. The average dose for an adult is 100 mg. When an optimal effect is obtained, reduction of the dosage with 2.5 mg every 4 weeks is started after 3–6 months. Necessary adjuncts include 80 to 120 mEq of potassium ion, antacids between meals, and a low-sodium, high-protein, low-carbohydrate diet [17]. Serial measurement of serum CPK activity is of great value in assessing the effects of treatment with corticosteroids [15]. Often the serum CPK activity returns to normal levels before an actual improvement of the muscular weakness is seen. On the other hand an increase of the CPK level may precede a clinical relapse, for instance when the rate of tapering off is too fast or the maintenance dose too low. When there is no improvement of muscle strength after 3–6 months of prednisone therapy, immunosuppressive drugs can be used. Methotrexate, azathioprine, cyclophosphamide, chlorambucil and 6-mercaptopurine [1, 5,20,30,31,35,36,44] have been given to these steroid resistant cases. So far, the series of patients treated with immunosuppressive drugs is relatively small, but good results were observed in many patients.

The dosage of prednisone necessary to control activity and progression of the disease is much smaller when combined with immunosuppressive drugs.

Adequate corticosteroid treatment is considered to be a major benefit in improving the degree of functional recovery of patients with polymyositis or dermatomyositis [15,37,42]. Other authors found improvement in only 20 per cent of their cases [35], while it has also been put forward that there is no conclusive evidence that either corticosteroids or immuno-suppressive drugs are effective in polymyositis and dermatomyositis [7]. A life table analysis revealed no difference in survivorship between males and females, between polymyositis and dermatomyositis or between those treated with or without corticosteroids [29].

Most authors agree that the prognosis is less favourable in patients with associated malignancy or collagen—vascular diseases.

References   1   Arnett,F.C.,Whelton,J.C.,Zizic,T.M.,Stevens,M.B.
                     Methotrexate therapy in polymyositis.
                     Ann.rheum.Dis.1973,32:536–546
             2   Banker,B.Q.
                     Dermatomyositis of childhood. Ultrastructural alterations of muscle and intramuscular blood vessels.
                     J.Neuropath.exp.Neurol.1975,34:46–75.
             3   Banker,B.Q.,Victor,M.
                     Dermatomyositis (systemic angiopathy) of childhood.
                     Medicine(Balt.)1966,45:261–289
             4   Bates,D.,Stevens,J.C.,Hudgson,P.
                     'Polymyositis' with involvement of facial and distal musculature. One form of the facioscapulohumeral syndrome?
                     J.neurol.Sci.1973,19:105–108

5   Benson,M.D.,Aldo,M.A.
     Azathioprine therapy in polymyositis.
     Arch.intern.Med.1973,132:547–551
6   Bohan,A.,Peter,J.B.
     Polymyositis and dermatomyositis (first of two parts).
     New Engl.J.Med.1975,292:344–347
7   Bohan,A.,Peter,J.B.
     Polymyositis and dermatomyositis (second of two parts).
     New Engl.J.Med.1975,292:403–407
8   Brooke,M.H.,Kaplan,H.
     Muscle pathology in rheumatoid arthritis, polymyalgia
     rheumatica and polymyositis.
     Arch.Path.1972,93:101–118
9   Camp,A.V.,Lane,D.J.,Mowat,A.G.
     Dermatomyositis with parenchymal lung involvement.
     Brit.med.J.1972,1:155–156
10   Carpenter,S.,Karpati,G.,Eisen,A.
     A morphologic study of muscle in polymyositis: clues to
     pathogenesis of different types.
     In:Recent Advances in Myology.Proceedings of the
     3rd International Congress on Muscle Diseases,Newcastle
     upon Tyne,15–21 September 1974.W.G.Bradley,
     D.Gardner-Medwin,J.N.Walton(eds.).Amsterdam,
     Excerpta Medica,1975,pp.374–379.(Int.Congr.Ser.360)
11   Chou,S.M.
     Myxovirus-like structures and accompanying nuclear changes
     in chronic polymyositis.
     Arch.Path.1968,86:649–658
12   Chou,S.M.,Gutmann,L.
     Picornavirus-like crystals in subacute polymyositis.
     Neurology(Minneap.)1970,20:205–213
13   Classification of the neuromuscular disorders.
     Appendix A to the minutes of the meeting of the Research
     Group on neuromuscular diseases, held in Montreal, Canada,
     on 21 September, 1967.
     J.neurol.Sci.1968,6:165–177
14   Currie,S.,Saunders,M.,Knowles,M.,Brown,A.E.
     Immunological aspects of polymyositis. The in vitro activity
     of lymphocytes on incubation with muscle antigen and
     with muscle cultures.

Quart.J.Med.1971,40:63–84
15   DeVere,R.,Bradley,W.G.
     Polymyositis: its presentation, morbidity and mortality.
     Brain 1975,98:637–666
16   Engel,W.K.,DeVivo,D.C.,Warmolts,J.R.,Schwartzman,R.J.
     High-single-dose alternate-day prednisone (HSDAD-PRED)
     in neuromuscular diseases.
     In:2nd International Congress on Muscle Diseases.
     Amsterdam,Excerpta Medica,1971,p.59.(Int.Congr.Ser.237)
17   Engel,W.K.,Askanas,V.
     Remote effects of focal cancer on the neuromuscular system.
     In:Advances in Neurology,Vol.15.R.A.Thompson,
     J.R.Green(eds.).NewYork,Raven Press,1976,pp.119–147
18   Fidziańska,A.
     Virus-like structures in muscle in chronic polymyositis.
     Acta neuropath.1973,23:23–31
19   Gotoff,S.P.,Smith,R.D.,Sugar,O.
     Dermatomyositis with cerebral vasculitis in a patient with
     agammaglobulinemia.
     Amer.J.Dis.Child.1972,123:53–56
20   Haas,D.C.
     Treatment of polymyositis with immunosuppressive drugs.
     Neurology(Minneap.)1973,23:55–62
21   Hughes,J.T.,Esiri,M.M.
     Ultrastructural studies in human polymyositis.
     J.neurol.Sci.1975,25:347–360
22   Johnson,R.L.,Fink,C.W.,Ziff,M.
     Lymphotoxin formation by lymphocytes and muscle in
     polymyositis.
     J.clin.Invest.1972,51:2435–2449
23   Krain,L.S.
     Dermatomyositis in six patients without initial muscle
     involvement.
     Arch.Derm.1975,111:241–245
24   Leddy,J.P.,Griggs,R.C.,Klemperer,M.R.,Frank,M.M.
     Hereditary complement (C2) deficiency with dermatomyositis.
     Amer.J.Med.1975,58:83–91
25   Martinez,A.J.,Hooshmand,H.,IndolosMendoza,G.,
     Winston,Y.E.

Fatal polymyositis: morphogenesis and ultrastructural features.
Acta neuropath.1974,29:251–262

26   Mastaglia,F.L.,Walton,J.N.
Coxsackie virus-like particles in skeletal muscle from
a case of polymyositis.
J.neurol.Sci.1970,11:593–599

27   Mastaglia,F.L.,Walton,J.N.
An ultrastructural study of skeletal muscle in polymyositis.
J.neurol.Sci.1971,12:473–504

28   MedsgerJr,T.A.,DawsonJr,W.N.,Masi,A.T.
The epidemiology of polymyositis.
Amer.J.Med.1970,48:715–723

29   MedsgerJr,T.A.,Robinson,H.,Masi,A.T.
Factors affecting survivorship in polymyositis. A life-table
study of 124 patients.
Arthr.andRheum.1971,14:249–258

30   Metzger,A.L.,Bohan,A.,Goldberg,L.S.,Bluestone,R.,
Pearson,C.M.
Polymyositis and dermatomyositis: combined methotrexate
and corticosteroid therapy.
Ann.intern.Med.1974,81:182–189

31   Mintz,G.,Fraga,A.,Valle,L.
Effect of immuno suppressive therapy in adult polymyositis.
In:Clinical Studies in Myology.Proceedings of the
2nd International Congress on Muscle Diseases,Perth,
22–26 November 1971,Part 2.B.A.Kakulas(ed.).
Amsterdam,Excerpta Medica,1973,pp.564–568.
(Int.Congr.Ser.295).

32   Munsat,T.,Cancilla,P.
Polymyositis without inflammation.
Bull.Los Angeles neurol.Soc.1974,39:113–120

33   Ozonoff,M.B.,FlynnJr,F.J.
Roentgenologic features of dermatomyositis of childhood.
Amer.J.Roentgenol.1973,118:206–212

34   Pearson,C.M.
Polymyositis.
Ann.Rev.Med.1966,17:63–82

35   Riddoch,D.,Morgan-Hughes,J.A.
Prognosis in adult polymyositis.

J.neurol.Sci.1975,26:71–80

36 Roget,J.,Rambaud,P.,Frappat,P.,Joannard,A.
Table ronde sur les collagénoses. La dermatomyosite
de l'enfant. Etude de 22 observations.
Pédiatrie 1971,26:471–490

37 Rose,A.L.,Walton,J.N.
Polymyositis: a survey of 89 cases with particular reference
to treatment and prognosis.
Brain 1966,89:747–768

38 Rothstein,T.L.,Carlson,C.B.,Sumi,S.M.
Polymyositis with facioscapulohumeral distribution.
Arch.Neurol.(Chic.)1971,25:313–319

39 Rowland,L.P.,Schotland,D.L.
Neoplasms and muscle disease.
In:The Remote Effects of Cancer on the Nervous System.
Lord Brain,F.H.Norris Jr(eds.).New York,Grune & Stratton,
1965,pp.83–97

40 Sato,T.,Walker,D.L.,Peters,H.A.,Reese,H.H.,Chou,S.M.
Chronic polymyositis and myxovirus-like inclusions. Electron
microscopic and viral studies.
Arch.Neurol.(Chic.)1971,24:409–418

41 Schwarz,M.I.,Matthay,R.A.,Sahn,S.A.,Stanford,R.E.,
Marmorstein,B.L.,Scheinhorn,D.J.
Interstitial lung disease in polymyositis and dermato-myositis:
analysis of six cases and review of the literature.
Medicine(Balt.)1976,55:89–104

42 Sullivan,D.B.,Cassidy,J.T.,Petty,R.E.,Burt,A.
Prognosis in childhood dermatomyositis.
J.Pediat.1972,80:555–563

43 Susac,J.O.,Garcia-Mullin,R.,Glaser,J.S.
Ophthalmoplegia in dermatomyositis.
Neurology(Minneap.)1973,23:305–310

44 Walton,J.N.
Polymyositis: new light on pathogenesis and treatment.
Proc.Aust.Ass.Neurol.1973,9:1–7

45 Walton,J.N.,Adams,R.D.
Polymyositis.
Edinburgh,Livingstone,1958

46   Whitaker,J.N.,Engel,W.K.
         Vascular deposits of immunoglobulin and complement in
         idiopathic inflammatory myopathy.
         New Engl.J.Med.1972,286:333–338
47   Yunis,E.J.,Samaha,F.J.
         Inclusion body myositis.
         Lab.Invest.1971,25:240–248

Muscle disorders associated with endocrine diseases

Neuromuscular disorders may be present in many diseases of the endocrine glands. In some cases, muscular weakness is the presenting symptom of the underlying endocrine disfunction and dominates the clinical picture. Knowledge of the possibility of the association of muscle involvement and endocrine disease is essential, as adequate treatment of the latter may result in full recovery of the muscular disorder.

Because the clinical muscular weakness is often of proximal distribution, and is associated with elevation of the serum creatine phosphokinase activity, creatinuria and short-duration low-amplitude motor unit potentials, this group of muscular disorders is usually referred to as endocrine myopathies. However, the myopathic caracter of the muscular manifestations is often uncertain, and there are many indications of its neuropathic nature [1–9].

References 1 Dyck,P.J.,Lambert,E.H.
Polyneuropathy associated with hypothyroidism.
J.Neuropath.exp.Neurol.1970,29:631–658

2 Feibel,J.H.,Campa,J.F.
Thyrotoxic neuropathy (Basedow's paraplegia).
J.Neurol.Neurosurg.Psychiat.1976,39:491–497

3 Havard,C.W.H.,Campbell,E.D.R.,Ross,H.B.,Spence,A.W.
Electromyographic and histological findings in the muscles
of patients with thyrotoxicosis.
Quart.J.Med.1963,32:145–163

4 Ludin,H.P.,Spiess,H.,Koenig,M.P.
Neuromuscular dysfunction associated with thyrotoxicosis.
Europ.Neurol.1969,2:269–278

5 Mallette,L.E.,Patten,B.M.,Engel,W.K.
Neuromuscular disease in secondary hyperparathyroidism.
Ann.intern.Med.1975,82:474–483

6 McComas,A.J.,Sica,R.E.P.,McNabb,A.R.,Goldberg,W.M.,
Upton,A.R.M.
Evidence for reversible motoneurone dysfunction in
thyrotoxicosis.
J.Neurol.Neurosurg.Psychiat.1974,37:548–558

7   Patten,B.M.,Bilezikian,J.P.,Mallette,L.E.,Prince,A.,
    Engel,W.K.,Aurbach,G.D.
    Neuromuscular disease in primary hyperparathyroidism.
    Ann.intern.Med.1974,80:182–193
8   Pleasure,D.E.,Walsh,G.O.,Engel,W.K.
    Atrophy of skeletal muscle in patients with Cushing's syndrome.
    Arch.Neurol.(Chic.)1970,22:118–125
9   Scarpalezos,S.,Lygidakis,C.,Papageorgiou,C.,Maliara,S.,
    Koukoulommati,A.S.,Koutras,D.A.
    Neural and muscular manifestations of hypothyroidism.
    Arch.Neurol.(Chic.)1973,29:140–144

Exophthalmic ophthalmoplegia is a well-known feature in thyroid over-activity. It is also called Graves' disease, endocrine exophthalmos or malignant exophthalmos; it is a self-limiting disease.

There is a weakness or complete paralysis of the external ocular muscles, especially of the muscles of upward gaze. In addition to diplopia, exophthalmos, chemosis and ptosis may be present. Exophthalmos may arise many months after successful treatment of thyrotoxicosis and, in fact, very severe exophthalmos may occur in the euthyroid state or in patients who have never had thyrotoxicosis [2]. Primary muscle pathology consists of interstitial inflammatory oedema.

Thyrotoxic myopathy. Chronic, mainly proximal muscular weakness, often associated with atrophy, is frequently present in thyrotoxicosis [8]. It may be the presenting symptom of hyperthyroidism [9] and predominate the clinical picture thus masking the underlying thyroid dysfunction. This muscle disorder can also occur in childhood [4]. The pathogenesis of the muscular weakness remains obscure.

Evidence of a myopathy has been shown by quantitative analytical electromyography [7]. A significantly reduced mean action potential duration was found in the proximal muscles in over 90 per cent of 54 consecutive, unselected patients with thyrotoxicosis. It has been postulated that the muscle weakness is attributed to reduced membrane excitability [1].

However, electromyographical evidence of a neuropathic process suggested the presence of sub-clinical polyneuropathy, predominantly involving the distal muscles of the legs [5]. Motor unit estimating techniques, carried out in 20 patients with thyrotoxicosis, showed evidence of reversible motoneurone disfunction in all patients [6].

Non-specific histopathological changes in the muscle were found in almost 70 per cent of 240 cases [9], but with the intravital methylene-blue staining technique, pathological changes in the terminal axons and end-plates were found in 27 of 35 patients [3], which is in favour of a neurogenic genesis of the muscular features.

Treatment of the hyperthyroidism results in complete recovery of the weakness.

Hypokalaemic periodic paralysis may be associated with thyrotoxicosis, especially in Oriental male patients (page 183).

Myasthenia gravis rarely developes in hyperthyroidism. On the other hand the incidence of hyperthyroidism in the course of myasthenia gravis constitutes approximately 5 per cent in most series.

References   1   Gruener,R.,Stern,L.Z.,Payne,C.,Hannapel,L.
                           Hyperthyroid myopathy. Intracellular electrophysiological
                           measurements in biopsied human intercostal muscle.
                           J.neurol.Sci.1975,24:339–349
                    2   Havard,C.W.H.
                           Endocrine exophthalmos.
                           Brit.med.J.1972,1:360–363
                    3   Havard,C.W.H.,Campbell,E.D.R.,Ross,H.B.,Spence,A.W.
                           Electromyographic and histological findings in the muscles
                           of patients with thyrotoxicosis.
                           Quart.J.Med.1963,32:145–163
                    4   Johnston,D.M.
                           Thyrotoxic myopathy.
                           Arch.Dis.Childh.1974,49:968–969
                    5   Ludin,H.P.,Spiess,H.,Koenig,M.P.
                           Neuromuscular dysfunction associated with thyrotoxicosis.
                           Europ.Neurol.1969,2:269–278
                    6   McComas,A.J.,Sica,R.E.P.,McNabb,A.R.,Goldberg,W.M.,
                           Upton,A.R.M.
                           Evidence for reversible motoneurone dysfunction in
                           thyrotoxicosis.
                           J.Neurol.Neurosurg.Psychiat.1974,37:548–558
                    7   Ramsay,I.D.
                           Electromyography in thyrotoxicosis.
                           Quart.J.Med.1965,34:255–267
                    8   Ramsay,I.D.
                           Muscle dysfunction in hyperthyroidism.
                           Lancet 1966,II:931–935

9   Satoyoshi,E.,Murakami,K.,Kowa,H.,Kinoshita,M.,Noguchi,K.,
Hoshina,S.,Nishiyama,Y.,Ito,K.
Myopathy in thyrotoxicosis. With special emphasis on an
effect of potassium ingestion on serum and urinary creatine.
Neurology(Minneap.)1963,13:645–658.

Hypothyroid myopathy and myxoedema myopathy are the names given to the muscular disorders in hypothyroidism. These are characterized by weakness, painful cramps, slowness of movements, muscular hypertrophy and, rarely, atrophy. The tendon reflexes are sluggish, which is best seen when the ankle jerks are elicted. In some patients, percussion of the muscle with a reflex hammer results in ridging of the muscle (myoedema). This phenomenon is also seen in other disorders such as cachexia and malabsorption and is therefore not specific for hypothyroidism. In contrast to percussion myotonia, it is electrically silent [4,10].

A marked raise of the serum creatine phosphokinase activity may be present.

Mild weakness of the proximal muscles of the legs and the extensors of the feet, without any other features, was considered to be due to a true myopathy [2].

The finding of a low acid maltase activity in the skeletal muscle of a patient with a myopathy associated with hypothyroidism [5], seems to be unrelated to the thyroid disfunction [6,7].

Kocher-Debré-Sémélaigne syndrome is the name that has been given to cretinous children with muscular hypertrophy (infant Hercules). There is slow relaxation of the tendon reflexes. Electromyography reveals brief and polyphasic motor unit potentials of small amplitude in most patients. Light and electron microscopic studies showed no or only non-specific changes, such as type I fibre atrophy, ringed fibres, focal accumulation of glycogen and mitochondrial aggregates [1,12]. These variable pathological findings may reflect variations in duration and degree of thyroid deficiency [12].

Hoffmann syndrome is the name that has been given to myxoedematous adults with muscular hypertrophy who also have painful spasms and abnormally slow contraction and relaxation of the muscles ('myotonoid' contraction or 'pseudomyotonia'). However, the Kocher-Debré-Sémélaigne syndrome and Hoffmann syndrome are considered by some authors as variants of the same disease process [8], and features of both syndromes may be encountered in children as well as in adults, or even in the course of hypothyroidism in the same patient. Muscle pathology in adults is non-specific, and includes ringed fibres and sarcoplasmic masses [9].

Neural manifestations. Polyneuropathy may develop in patients with hypothyroidism, but the muscular weakness is usually mild. Abnormalities of motor conduction, consisting of a prolonged distal latency and a slowing of the motor conduction velocity, may be found [11].
In teased-fibre studies, segmental demyelination and remyelination were demonstrated [3].
Some patients complain of paraesthesias of the extremities. Entrapment of the median nerve at the wrist (carpal tunnel syndrome) is a well-known complication of myxoedema.

Myasthenic syndromes in hypothyroidism are rare [13], although hypo-thyroidism may develop more frequently in patients with myasthenia gravis.

References   1   Afifi,A.K.,Najjar,S.S.,Mire-Salman,J.,Bergman,R.A.
                  The myopathology of the Kocher-Debré-Sémélaigne
                  syndrome. Electromyography, light- and
                  electron-microscopic study.
                  J.neurol.Sci.1974,22:445–470
              2   Astrom,K.-E.,Kugelberg,E.,Muller,R.
                  Hypothyroid myopathy.
                  Arch.Neurol.(Chic.)1961,5:472–482
              3   Dyck,P.J.,Lambert,E.H.
                  Polyneuropathy associated with hypothyroidism.
                  J.Neuropath.exp.Neurol.1970,29:631–658
              4   Giménez-Roldán,S.,Esteban,A.
                  Orbicularis 'myotonia' in hypothyroid myopathy.
                  Europ.Neurol.1973,9:44–55

5   Hurwitz,L.J.,McCormick,D.,Allen,I.V.
     Reduced muscle-glucosidase (acid-maltase) activity in
     hypothyroid myopathy.
     Lancet 1970,1:67–69

6   Koster,J.F.
     Acid-maltase activity and hypothyroidism.
     Lancet 1970,II:1187

7   McCormick,D.,Allen,I.V.,Hurwitz,L.J.
     Acid-maltase activity and hypothyroidism.
     Lancet 1971,I:85–86

8   NorrisJr,F.H.,Panner,B.J.
     Hypothyroid myopathy. Clinical, electromyographical and
     ultrastructural observations.
     Arch.Neurol.(Chic.)1966,14:574–589

9   Roger,P.,Coquet,M.,LeBlanc,M.,Vital,C.,Latapie,J.-L.,
     Rivière,J.
     Un cas de myopathie hypothyroïdienne: étude ultrastructurale.
     Sem.Hôp.Paris.1973,49:1765–1768

10   Salick,A.I.,ColachisJr,S.C.,Pearson,C.M.
     Myxedema myopathy: clinical, electrodiagnostic, and
     pathologic findings in advanced case.
     Arch.phys.med.Rehab.1968,49:230–237

11   Scarpalezos,S.,Lygidakis,C.,Papageorgiou,C.,Maliara,S.,
     Koukoulommati,A.S.,Koutras,D.A.
     Neural and muscular manifestations of hypothyroidism.
     Arch.Neurol.(Chic.)1973,29:140–144

12   Spiro,A.J.,Hirano,A.,Beilin,R.L.,Finkelstein,J.W.
     Cretinism with muscular hypertrophy (Kocher-Debré-
     Sémélaigne syndrome). Histochemical and ultrastructural
     study of skeletal muscle.
     Arch.Neurol.(Chic.)1970,23:340–349

13   Takamori,M.,Gutmann,L.,Crosby,T.W.,Martin,J.D.
     Myasthenic syndromes in hypothyroidism. Electrophysiological
     study of neuromuscular transmission and muscle
     contraction in two patients.
     Arch.Neurol.(Chic.)1972,26:326–335

In primary and secondary hyperparathyroidism, easy fatigability and weakness of the proximal muscles are frequently present [1]. In disorders in which osteomalacia may develop, e.g. intestinal malabsorption, gastric resections and renal tubular defects, these muscular complaints may constitute the presenting symptoms and thus simulate a primary myopathic syndrome [13].

The name osteomalacic myopathy has been used for these muscular disorders. Nutritional osteomalacia has been observed especially in India [5], but may be seen in other countries in patients taking inadequate diets [7]. Hypophosphataemic osteomalacia and myopathy may develop in patients who are treated with aluminium hydroxide [2,6].

Usually the first symptom is a feeling of heaviness in the legs and painful discomfort after muscular exercise. This is followed by proximal muscle weakness of the legs, while involvement of the muscles of the trunk and arms (especially the abductors) tends to occur later. There is no correlation of the degree of muscular involvement and the levels of serum calcium or phosphorus. Severe bone pain may often lead to considerable difficulty in testing muscular function and evaluating muscular weakness. The muscles can become atrophic, but serum creatine phosphokinase activity is usually normal. Generally, the tendon reflexes are hyper-active. Babinski's sign was found in many patients with primary hyperparathyroidism [9]. Other clinical features are pressure tenderness of the bones [4,13] and mental symptoms.

The finding of decreased vibration sensation, abnormal movements of the tongue — resembling fasciculations — the presence of signs of denervation on electromyography and of angular atrophic muscle fibres, especially type II fibres, in biopsies, are in favour of a neuropathic nature of the muscular features [8,9].

In one case, both type I and type II fibres had a high phosphorylase activity with otherwise normal histochemical differentiation of the two fibre types [3].

Ultrastructural studies of the muscle in osteomalacia due to malnutrition revealed atrophic fibres without any degenerative changes. The latter were present, however, when the patients suffered from other metabolic or endocrinological disorders, in addition to malnutrition [5].

The neuromuscular disorder in primary hyperparathyroidism can be treated by removal of the tumour, usually an adenoma. In patients with osteomalacia and secondary hyperparathyroidism, there is a favourable response to treatment with vitamin D [11,12]. In primary hypophosphataemic osteomalacia in adults, the myopathy can be cured by vitamin D therapy without affecting the hypophosphataemia [10,12]. In iatrogenic hypophosphataemic osteomalacia with myopathy, both features can be cured by correction of the hypophosphataemia without vitamin D therapy [2,6].

References   1   Aurbach,G.D.,Mallette,L.E.,Patten,B.M.,Heath,D.A.,
Doppman,J.L.,Bilezikian,J.P.
Hyperparathyroidism: recent studies.
Ann.intern.Med.1973,79:566–581

2   Baker,L.R.I.,Ackrill,P.,Cattell,W.R.,Stamp,T.C.B.,Watson,L.
Iatrogenic osteomalacia and myopathy due to phosphate
depletion.
Brit.med.J.1974,3:150–152

3   Cape,C.A.
Increased phosphorylase activity in muscle in hyperparathyroid
disease.
Neurology(Minneap.)1971,21:638–641

4   Cholod,E.J.,Haust,M.D.,Hudson,A.J.,Lewis,F.N.
Myopathy in primary familial hyperparathyroidism.
Clinical and morphologic studies.
Amer.J.Med.1970,48:700–707

5   Dastur,D.K.,Gagrat,B.M.,Wadia,N.H.,Desai,M.M.,
Bharucha,E.P.
Nature of muscular change in osteomalacia: light- and
electron microscope observations.
J.Path.1975,117:211–228

6   Dent,C.E.,Winter,C.S.
Osteomalacia due to phosphate depletion from excessive
aluminium hydroxide ingestion.
Brit.med.J.1974,1:551–552

7   Gough,K.R.,Lloyd,O.C.,Wills,M.R.
    Nutritional osteomalacia.
    Lancet 1964,II:1261–1264
8   Mallette,L.E.,Patten,B.M.,Engel,W.K.
    Neuromuscular disease in secondary hyperparathyroidism.
    Ann.intern.Med.1975,82:474–483
9   Patten,B.M.,Bilezikian,J.P.,Mallette,L.E.,Prince,A.,
    Engel,W.K.,Aurbach,G.D.
    Neuromuscular disease in primary hyperparathyroidism.
    Ann.intern.Med.1974,80:182–193
10 Schott,G.D.,Wills,M.R.
    Myopathy in hypophosphataemic osteomalacia presenting
    in adult life.
    J.Neurol.Neurosurg.Psychiat.1975,38:297–304
11 Smith,R.,Stern,G.
    Myopathy, osteomalacia and hyperparathyroidism.
    Brain 1967,90:593–602
12 Smith,R.,Stern,G.
    Muscular weakness in osteomalacia and hyperparathyroidism.
    J.neurol.Sci.1969,8:511–520
13 Vicale,C.T.
    The diagnostic features of a muscular syndrome resulting
    from hyperparathyroidism, osteomalacia owing to renal
    tubular acidosis, and perhaps to related disorders of calcium
    metabolism.
    Trans.Amer.neurol.Ass.1949,74:143–147

Muscle disorders in acromegaly

There may be muscular hypertrophy in the early stages of acromegaly. In a later stage of the disease, many patients complain of fatigue and muscular weakness. In some patients, evidence of a myopathy was found [2,5], with mild proximal muscle weakness, elevation of the serum creatine phosphokinase activity and short duration of motor unit potentials. Light and electron microscopic studies revealed non-specific changes in the muscle biopsies, including tubular aggregates [4]. The occurrence of poly-neuropathy, carpal tunnel syndrome, vocal cord fixation and nerve root lesions have also been described [2].

Muscle disorders in Cushing syndrome

Cushing syndrome is often associated with muscular weakness and wasting. The paresis is most pronounced in the proximal muscles of the legs, but the muscles of the shoulder girdle and the extensors of the feet may also be involved [7].

The weakness may appear several years after the onset of the disease. Muscle wasting was found to be due to profound atrophy of muscle fibres, mainly of the type II fibres [9,10].

Although bilateral total adrenalectomy may result in complete recovery of the muscular symptoms [3,9], treatment of the Cushing syndrome had no, or only slight, effect on the muscular features in another series [7].

Following treatment of Cushing syndrome by adrenalectomy and sub-sequent replacement steroid therapy, development of pigmentation of the skin has been reported together with excessive muscle fatigue on effort and mild proximal weakness or bilateral ptosis [10]. Muscle biopsy showed excessive subsarcolemmal accumulation of lipid in both fibre types.

Acute development of a polyneuropathy was observed in the post-operative period in a patient who had undergone adrenalectomy for Cushing syndrome [12].

Steroid myopathy

Proximal muscular weakness and wasting may develop in patients under treatment with corticosteroids [6,8]. This is associated with creatinuria and a decrease in the duration of the motor unit potentials. Muscle biopsy shows selective type II fibre atrophy and, at the ultrastructural level, collections of enlarged and abnormal mitochondria and subsarcolemmal accumulation of glycogen. Withdrawal of the drug results in complete recovery of the muscular weakness and atrophy.

Muscle disorders in Addison's disease
Addison's disease is often associated with progressive asthenia and fatigue. In some patients, muscle cramps and contractures may be seen. When hyperkalaemia is present, attacks of flaccid paralysis, predominantly involving the distal parts of the lower extremities, can occur [1].

Muscle disorders in primary hyperaldosteronism
Primary hyperaldosteronism or Conn syndrome can give rise to periodic attacks of muscular weakness due to the marked renal loss of potassium (page 183). Persistent and progressive proximal muscular weakness and wasting, with a high activity of serum creatine phosphokinase, were present in a patient who also showed electromyographical and histopathological alterations, thought to be consistent with a myopathy. Removal of an adrenal adenoma resulted in a full recovery of the muscular disorder [11].

References **1** Duc,M.,Duc,M.L.,Mauuary,G.
Paralysies intermittentes pas hyperkalémie révèlatrices
d'une maladie d'Addison.
Ann.méd.Nancy,1970,9:387–390
2 Lundberg,P.O.,Osterman,P.O.,Stålberg,E.
Neuromuscular signs and symptoms in acromegaly.
In:Muscle Diseases.Proceedings of an International Congress,
Milan,19–21May,1969.J.N.Walton,N.Canal,G.Scarlato(eds.).
Amsterdam,Excerpta Medica,1970,pp.531–534
3 Luton,J.P.,Valcke,J.C.,Turpin,G.,Forest,M.,Bricaire,H.
Muscle et syndrome de Cushing.
Ann.Endocr.(Paris)1971,32:157–169

4 Mastaglia,F.L.
Pathological changes in skeletal muscle in acromegaly.
Acta neuropath.1973,24:273–286

5 Mastaglia,F.L.,Barwick,D.D.,Hall,R.
Myopathy in acromegaly.
Lancet 1970,II:907–909

6 Moser,H.,Fiechter,R.,Ludin,H.P.,Jerusalem,F.
Die Steroidmyopathie im Kindesalter.
Z.Kinderheilk.1974,118:177–196

7 Müller,R.,Kugelberg,E.
Myopathy in Cushing's syndrome.
J.Neurol.Neurosurg.Psychiat.1959,22:314–319

8 Perkoff,G.T.,Silber,R.,Tyler,F.H.,Cartwright,G.E.,
Wintrobe,M.M.
Studies in disorders of muscle. XII. Myopathy due to be
administration of therapeutic amounts of
17-hydroxycorticosteroids.
Amer.J.Med.1959,26:891–898

9 Pleasure,D.E.,Walsh,G.O.,Engel,W.K.
Atrophy of skeletal muscle in patients with Cushing's
syndrome.
Arch.Neurol.(Chic.)1970,22:118–125

10 Prineas,J.,Hall,R.,Barwick,D.D.,Watson,A.J.
Myopathy associated with pigmentation following
adrenalectomy for Cushing's syndrome.
Quart.J.Med.1968,37:63–77

11 Sambrook,M.A.,Heron,J.R.,Aber,G.M.
Myopathy in association with primary hyperaldosteronism.
J.Neurol.Neurosurg.Psychiat.1972,35:202–207

12 Schindler,H.,Koller,K.
Schwere Myopathie und periphere Nervenläsion bei
Cushing-Syndrom infolge eines Nebennierenrindenadenoms.
Wien.med.Wschr.1974,51:758–761

Other muscle disorders

There are a few reports on the development of muscular weakness several years after the first symptoms of a carcinoid. Generalized wasting and weakness, fasciculations, muscular tenderness and distal paraesthesias, have been described [2], while mainly proximal muscle weakness and wasting were found by other authors [1,3]. Electromyography revealed short-duration, low-amplitude, polyphasic motor unit potentials, without evidence of denervation.

Muscle biopsy showed an increased variability of the diameter of both fibre types, an increased number of fibres with central nuclei, and type II fibre atrophy.

It has been suggested that carcinoid myopathy may be due to excess circulating serotonin (5-HT). In two patients, there was an increase of the urinary 5-hydroxyindoleacetic acid (5-HIAA) excretion [1,3], while in one the blood serotonin concentration was markedly raised [1]. These patients showed an improvement of the muscular weakness following treatment with cyproheptadine hydrochloride, a serotonin antagonist.

References   1   Berry,E.M.,Maunder,C.,Wilson,M.
                  Carcinoid myopathy and treatment with cyproheptadine
                  (Periactin).
                  Gut 1974,15:34–38
             2   Green,D.,Joynt,R.J.,VanAllen,M.W.
                  Neuromyopathy associated with a malignant carcinoid tumor.
                  A case report.
                  Arch.intern.Med.1964,114:494–496
             3   Swash,M.,Fox,K.P.,Davidson,A.R.
                  Carcinoid myopathy. Serotonin-induced muscle weakness
                  in man?
                  Arch.Neurol.(Chic.)1975,32:572–574

Xanthine oxidase catalyses the oxidation of hypoxanthine to xanthine and of xanthine to uric acid. Xanthine oxidase deficiency is a rare hereditary disorder of purine metabolism, in which there is marked hypouricaemia with increased amounts of xanthine and hypoxanthine in the blood and urine.

Muscular complaints, such as slight muscular weakness, muscle pain [4] cramp-like pain or discomfort on exercise [2,3] have been reported in this disease. Also arthralgia and tenderness of muscle on pressure were described [1].

In one case, many polyphasic motor unit potentials of short duration were found on electromyography [2]. Muscle biopsies were normal [4] or showed an unusually high average diameter of the muscle fibres and an increased number of centrally placed nuclei [2]. In the muscle tissue hypoxanthine and xanthine crystals were seen [1,3]. The presence of xanthine and of increased amounts of hypoxanthine was also demonstrated by high resolution mass spectrometry. In muscle extracts, the level of xanthine plus hypoxanthine was found to be markedly elevated.

References   1   Berman,L.,Solomon,L.
'Xanthine gout'. Crystal deposition in skeletal muscle in a case of xanthinuria.
Rhumatologie(Paris)1975,5:253–256

2   Chalmers,R.A.,Johnson,M.,Pallis,C.,Watts,R.W.E.
Xanthinuria with myopathy (with some observations on the renal handling of oxypurines in the disease).
Quart.J.Med.1969,38:493–512

3   Chalmers,R.A.,Watts,R.W.E.,Bitensky, L., Chayen,J.
Microscopic studies on crystals in skeletal muscle from two cases of xanthinuria.
J.Path.1969,99:45–56

4   Isaacs,H.,Heffron,J.J.A.,Berman,L.,Badenhorst,M.,
Pickering,A.
Xanthine, hypoxanthine and muscle pain. Histochemical and biochemical observations.
S.Afr.med.J.1975,49:1035–1038

In 1969 Brody [1] described a 26—year-old male with muscle stiffness during exercise.

No abnormality was noted at birth and the motor milestones were normal. He first complained at the age of 5 years. After that painless muscle stiffness occurred during vigorous exercise or on sudden, rapid movements. The stiffness disappeared completely after 5–15 seconds of rest. He was able to carry out daily activities, including sport, without difficulty. Muscle stiffness occurred more readily in cold weather. There was no progression of the condition. He had no episodes of myoglobinuria.

Examination revealed no muscular weakness or wasting. The muscles showed a progressive slowing of relaxation with vigorous exercise. After repetitive contraction with maximal effort, the muscle became paralysed in a state of marked shortening.

Serum creatine phosphokinase activity was normal. Venous lactate at rest was elevated, but there was a normal rise after ischaemic forearm exercise. Neither the rate of development nor the severity of the muscle stiffness was altered by ischaemia, but they were increased after the patient had been three minutes in a cold room ($-5\,^{\circ}C$).

Motor nerve conduction velocities were normal.

Electromyography was normal. The shortened muscles showed no electrical activity, as is seen in true contracture.

Isometric tension myograms of the adductor pollicis muscle during voluntary contraction revealed a normal contraction phase, but there was a prolongation of the relaxation phase.

Light and electron microscopy of a muscle biopsy did not disclose any abnormalities.

On biochemical assay muscle glycogen content and the activities of phosphoglucomutase and alpha-glucosidase were normal. The total phosphorylase activity was normal but there was an abnormally high proportion (92 per cent) of active phosphorylase.

There was a marked decrease in the ability of the isolated sarcoplasmic reticulum to accumulate calcium ions. It has been suggested that after strong voluntary contraction the sarcoplasmic reticulum may not be able to reaccumulate the calcium rapidly. This gives rise to a persistently high level of calcium in the aqueous sarcoplasm, prolonging the mechanical shortening of the myofibrils. As calcium ions activate phosphorylase b kinase, which converts inactive to active phosphorylase, the high percentage of active phosphorylase in the patient's muscle may also be explained by the high concentration of calcium. The high level of blood lactate during rest was explained by the persistent activation of muscle phosphorylase.

The disease was thus thought to be attributable to a selective defect of a relaxing factor, i.e. the ability of the sarcoplasmic reticulum to accumulate calcium.

In 1972, Sreter, Bauman, Gergely and Luca [2] reported on a 16-year-old male with muscle stiffness and pain after exercise.

Birth and developmental milestones were normal. The patient first complained at the age of 12 years, when he experienced aching and stiffness in the muscles of the legs during vigorous exercise.

On examination the muscles appeared to be normal in contour, bulk, strength and tone. The symptoms, which were elicited by letting the patient run up and down several flights of stairs, disappeared after 30 seconds of rest.

Serum creatine phosphokinase activity was normal. There was a normal rise of venous lactate after ischaemic forearm exercise.

Electromyography was normal and no electrical activity was seen during the periods of muscle stiffness.

Light and electron microscopy of a muscle biopsy revealed no abnormalities. Biochemical assays showed a low creatine phosphate level, a low myosin ATPase activity and a high calcium uptake — in both extent and rate — by the fragmented sarcoplasmic reticulum. Glycolytic enzymes, muscle glycogen and phosphorylase activity were normal. It was not apparent in what way these biochemical abnormalities were related to the clinical features.

References 1 Brody,I.A.
Muscle contracture induced by exercise. A syndrome
attributable to decreased relaxing factor.
New Engl.J.Med.1969,281:187–192
2 Sreter,F.A.,Bauman,M.L.,Gergely,J.,Luca,N.
Changes in muscle chemistry associated with stiffness
and pain.
Neurology(Minneap.)1972,22:1172–1175